"The Greatest Good to the Greatest Number"

American University Studies

Series IX
History

Vol. 93

PETER LANG
New York • Bern • Frankfurt am Main • Paris

David P. Adams

"The Greatest Good to the Greatest Number"

Penicillin Rationing on the American Home Front, 1940-1945

PETER LANG
New York • Bern • Frankfurt am Main • Paris

Library of Congress Cataloging-in-Publication Data

Adams, David P. (David Parrish)
 "The greatest good to the greatest number" :
penicillin rationing on the American home front,
1940-1945 / David P. Adams.
   p. cm. — (American university studies. Series IX,
History ; vol. 93)
   Includes bibliographical references.
   1. Penicillin—Government policy—United States—
History. 2. Rationing, Consumer—Government
policy—United States—History. 3. Medical policy—
United States—History. I. Title. II. Series.
RM666.P35A33   1991   362.1′783—dc20   90-6081
ISBN 0-8204-1284-8   CIP
ISSN 0740-0462

© Peter Lang Publishing, Inc., New York 1991

All rights reserved.
Reprint or reproduction, even partially, in all forms such as microfilm,
xerography, microfiche, microcard, offset strictly prohibited.

Printed in the United States of America.

Table of Contents

Preface vii

Introduction 1

Chapter One   "Medical Preparedness" 25

Chapter Two   Out of the Ivory Tower 45

Chapter Three   "The Greatest Good to the Greatest Number"   65

Chapter Four   A "Rush on Penicillin" 103

Chapter Five   The Office of Civilian Penicillin Distribution ... 131

Chapter Six   The Legacy of Wartime Penicillin Rationing ... 153

Conclusion 185

Table 3-1 193

Bibliography 195

Index 221

Preface

Penicillin stands as an idol of the postwar baby boom generation. Few Americans born since 1945 have remained untouched by this drug in some way. Thousands of individuals receive penicillin each day for infections, while many have developed allergies to it. Others have had their children dosed with the drug.

This book is about penicillin, "the wonder drug of 1943," but it is also a study of persons who came face to face with bureaucracy, the authority of the American medical establishment, and a coolly objective rationing system. This system could function as a beneficent provider of a life-saving drug or as a cruel reminder of the power of the State. Abstractions such as fairness, equitability, or, as one clinician noted, "the greatest good to the greatest number" held little comfort to the seriously ill who believed that only penicillin could save them. Today, Americans suffering from scratchy throats, coughs, and fevers continue to see their physicians in search of penicillin or similar antibiotic to "cure" their ills. The "mystique" of penicillin remains decades after the introduction of the drug.

Although the results of this study are my responsibility alone, a number of individuals read the manuscript and offered invaluable comments. I particularly would like to thank my doctoral advisor, Prof. Kermit L. Hall, Professors Frederick Gregory, Lee Crandall, Harry Marks, and John Patrick Swann; and Dr. Kenneth M. Ludmerer, who initially encouraged me to pursue the topic of penicillin on the American home front as a seminar paper at Washington University in St. Louis. Daniel T. Savett, Drew Amery, Monica Hupalo, and James Riddle provided invaluable research assistance. Melanie Oyster was also of enormous help in proofreading the manuscript. The American Institute of the History of Pharmacy generously provided a grant-in-aid that funded the dissertation on which this study is based. Most of all, I would like to thank my wife, Teri, for her patience during the completion of this project. She, perhaps more than any other person, is glad the book is finished.

Introduction

This book deals with a sequence of events now more than forty years in the past: the rationing of penicillin during the Second World War. The distribution of this "wonder drug" reveals a great deal about wartime America, but it also holds important lessons about how contemporary policy makers might distribute medical resources more equitably. This study does not purport to be an examination of penicillin's development or production. Those aspects of the drug's history have received careful study elsewhere. My purpose lies in an examination of penicillin's clinical investigation and, by definition, the rationing decisions that had an impact upon the drug's use.[1]

The word "rationing" holds negative connotations for many Americans (especially those who lived through the Second World War), because it brings to mind wartime crises and shortages. However, "rationing," in the case of wartime penicillin, represents a better alternative than "allocating" since the former connotes equitable distribution rather than the simple apportionment of a commodity during times of scarcity. As this study will suggest, clinicians and policymakers provided penicillin to civilian patients in an extremely equitable manner.[2]

Because of the social value placed upon personal health, the concept of nonmarket rationing disturbs many Americans. Access to medical care, they believe, is much too important to be left to impersonal decision-making. Far better that one has access to health care through the free market system. Rationing also produces Orwellian images of a "centralized, impersonal, and arbitrary authority" wielded by a "central czar." "People," Mary Ann Baily remarked, "fear the situation in which they will feel they need a certain kind of care to survive, and a faraway bureaucrat, who can't be reasoned with, will have decided they can't have it." Access to health care on the free market, despite its bias in favor of the economically advantaged and well-insured, removes that threat.[3]

The concept of nonmarket rationing also disturbs many Americans because historically the United States has relied upon the free market to distribute resources. One's access to health care, therefore, has typically rested upon one's ability (or an insurer's) to pay for treatment. Market-regulated distribution, however, has exhibited sinister results on occasion, as Graham Greene's *The Third Man* described so vividly. The scarcity of penicillin in postwar Europe—scarce for civilians, that is—created a booming black market that Harry Lyme exploited by selling the adulterated drug to ailing individuals. His greed resulted in numerous deaths, including those of young children. Lyme displayed little remorse; this was for him a business decision.[4]

The grim scenario depicted in *The Third Man* highlights the limits of free market distribution: 1) only persons with financial resources receive treatment and 2) even if one can afford treatment, that treatment may not be efficacious. Even insured patients (who lack the funds to pay for a procedure) may not receive treatment because of the refusal of some companies to reimburse them for therapy considered "experimental." Institutional ethics committees may debate competing claims for a particular therapy, but the mere *cost* of a particular treatment may exclude some individuals from receiving any consideration at all. Postwar medicine, thus, has created a demand for a level of health care from which not all can reap benefits.[5]

Free market distribution, therefore, forces individuals to pay for their own care, make media pitches for funds, or receive no care at all. Some individuals plead for money to offset the cost of bone marrow transplants, others seek a donor organ. The successful individual often is the one who has attracted the most media coverage. Others, unable to touch the public's heartstrings, remain without the necessary financial and/or medical resources.[6]

The media have played an important role in helping patients gain access to one of the scarcest of all medical resources, transplant organs. "Baby Jesse," previously denied a donor heart, received a transplant following her parents' appearance on *Donahue* in June 1986. The Loma Linda Medical Center initially had refused little Jesse on the grounds that her unmarried parents would be unable to understand fully the child's complicated postoperative treatment program. The child received the heart, not through the national organ donor network but from a private source.[7]

Without media exposure, Baby Jesse might never have received the organ transplant. The parents of the brain-dead infant who donated their child's heart to Baby Jesse admitted that television reports had influenced their decision. A Louisville, Kentucky, infant (who had waited even longer for a donor heart), however, had been denied the organ that Jesse received. The parents of this child—unlike those of Baby Jesse—had sought a donor organ through conventional transplant networks. When they learned that Baby Jesse had circumvented the usual selection process, they retorted that "it almost seems like publicity is the only method that's working." Senator Albert Gore added his own pointed commentary: "What do we tell families, that they have to go on the Phil Donahue Show [to be considered]?"[8]

Emotion-charged media appeals obscure the medical criteria by which patients might be selected. Persons who are least likely to survive might receive media attention—and thereby acquire the desired therapy—while more favorable candidates might be ignored. Moreover, the health care system may yield to public pressure and distribute its resources to the darling of the nightly news broadcast. "It is not uncommon for medical decisions not to treat," political scientist Robert Blank has noted, "to be reversed by public outcry over the denial." The media have created "a circus-like atmosphere" complete with talk show appearances and press conferences, he added. Indeed, reporters often focus on the most dramatic cases, leaving the less newsworthy patients to seek aid from conventional sources. Those individuals who cannot attract a donor or funds through the media receive no care.[9]

Treatments such as kidney dialysis or organ or marrow transplantation generate huge medical bills—often not covered by insurance because the therapy is considered "experimental." Ronnie De-

Silliers, a seven-year-old liver transplant patient, generated hospital bills of more than $400,000 before he died in April 1987. Another child, three-year-old Tabatha Foster of Pittsburgh, had accrued medical bills of more than $250,000. Joe Williams, a lawyer who had sought funds for the little girl, lamented the inequity of a system that turned upon one's ability to pay for treatment. Bioethicist Arthur Caplan offered his own observation, "Do we want to give access to this type of operation based on ability to pay, and make the recipients pay for it? The obvious answer is yes, because we do."[10]

The donor organ market has boomed in recent years with an unanticipated result. *The Hastings Center Report* noted in 1984 that while some 10,000 Americans awaited transplant kidneys three hundred organs instead sold for top dollar to patients in Great Britain, Kuwait, Japan, and Turkey. American companies such as the South-Eastern Organ Procurement Foundation of Richmond, Virginia, and American Medical International, based in Hollywood, California, have masterminded the export of these organs while telling unsuspecting donors that fellow Americans would receive them. Moreover, Pittsburgh's Presbyterian Hospital gave priority to sixty-one wealthy foreigners who sought transplants. Deference to the children of physicians and government officials, hospital spokespersons explained, had influenced their decisions. The *Hastings Center Report* noted, however, that contrary to official hospital statements "money played a major role in the decision." The sixty-one patients treated at Presbyterian Hospital had paid a total of $427,000 in surgical fees—almost four times as much per operation as an American patient. One estimate has suggested that over 1,200 foreign patients had received American kidneys in the eighteen months between mid-1984 and early 1986 alone.[11]

The donor organ market has reached even more grotesque proportions. Japanese loan sharks, for example, allow debtors to repay them in kidneys instead of cash, while Philippine prisoners exchange kidneys for early paroles. In Bombay, a woman sold one of her kidneys for seven thousand dollars—to raise money for her daughter's dowry, a clock, a television, and a swivel fan. The donor organ market has even become a fertile field for unscrupulous fund-raisers. One Washington, D.C., rock music promoter solicited individuals desperate for an organ donor and had a nineteen-year-old mother offer him $10,000 dollars to raise funds for her baby's transplant. In Virginia, a physician-turned-entrepreneur declared himself an organ broker and acquired a license to import organs from foreign countries. Another individual even tried to place his liver on the open market, stopping short when he realized the fatal implications of such an act.[12]

Free-market rationing of medical resources, with or without media assistance, favors persons most able to pay for therapy. How, then, can health care be distributed more equitably? Dr. Felix T. Rapaport of the State University of New York at Stony Brook has suggested that medical criteria alone should determine distribution of scarce medical resources. Rapaport voiced particular concern over the abundance of "sensational news coverage" and a growing tendency "to inject shrill political philosophies into what should remain strictly medical guidelines for patient treatment—a direct intrusion into the doctor-patient relationship." Race, religion, or political affiliation, he commented, have no place in transplant decisions, and the medical profession must resist these trends. "The potential distortion of such criteria by political prejudice or the establishment of priorities on the basis of socioeconomic criteria ...," Rapaport concluded, "are a particularly repugnant aspect of the present situation [in scarce medical resource distribution]." He especially disliked "the bureaucratic alternative of having huge numbers of ... organs flying back and forth in the American skies before they are ever implanted into recipients selected by a distant national bureau."[13]

Rapaport correctly assessed the efficacy of distribution according to medical criteria. Investigators have recently carried out AZT trials, for example, by such means. He underestimated, however, the ability of bureaucracy to ration medical resources equitably. During the Second World War, the Committee on Chemotherapeutic and Other Agents (hereafter referred to as the COC or the Committee on Chemotherapy, a term used by the wartime press) distributed penicillin in a manner that avoided lay influence while effectively employing bureaucratic rationing techniques. The Committee functioned as an efficient bureaucratic organization rather than the malevolent "national bureau" which Rapaport described. The COC used bureaucracy to insure that deserving civilian patients enjoyed equal access to penicillin.[14]

Nor did penicillin distribution fall prey to the dangers of political pressures that so concerned Rapaport. Rationing the drug, COC Chairman Chester Keefer attempted to maintain strict impartiality despite attempts by a wide range of individuals to sway the Committee's decisions. While the COC distributed penicillin, even financial issues did not influence rationing, since the government supplied the drug free of charge to civilian patients. Only after the Office of Civilian Penicillin Distribution (OCPD) had taken responsibility for penicillin rationing (leaving the COC to concentrate on clinical investigation) did patients actually pay for treatment with the drug.[15]

The socio-political context in which penicillin rationing occurred influenced the manner by which the COC distributed the drug. The penicillin effort took place in an era which, according to historian William Polenberg, "redefined" relations between individuals and the government. Barry Karl has added that wartime Americans faced an increased presence of government in their lives as the federal bureaucracy expanded to direct everything from gasoline rationing to the internment of Japanese-Americans.[16]

The war years also represented an important period in the growth of government-supported scientific and medical research. As A. Hunter Dupree's *Science in the Federal Government* noted, the creation of the National Defense Research Committee (NDRC) in 1940 represented a critical watershed in the history of the relationship between the federal government and university-based researchers. A strong alliance was forged that same year between the National Research Council's Division of Medical Sciences and the Armed Forces. The next year the Roosevelt Administration created the Office of Scientific Research and Development (OSRD) and the Committee on Medical Research (CMR), the agency which contracted the COC to conduct the clinical investigation of penicillin. The war years initiated an "exponential growth" in the number of researchers in the service of scientific and medical policy making.[17]

The development of penicillin stands as an integral part of the wartime research effort. The evolution of "science's Cinderella" from laboratory curiosity to mass-produced "wonder drug" has made it an especially alluring topic. Contemporary accounts, biographical studies of Alexander Fleming and Howard Florey, and histories of penicillin's industrial production appeared as early as the final years of the war. However, a detailed analysis of the wartime policy of civilian penicillin rationing has yet to appear.[18]

A study of the rationing of the drug to American civilians reveals a complex interaction of national defense interests, the professional authority of American academic physicians, and wartime bureaucracy. The penicillin effort influenced the relationship between academic researchers and the federal government as well as the role of physicians in postwar American society. Far removed from the Oxford labs, the Peoria pilot plants, and the pioneering clinical studies conducted by the nation's leading clinicians also existed the issue of providing the drug for ill civilians. Home-front Americans, perhaps, represented the most poignant aspect of wartime penicillin distribution, for they were the individuals who sometimes lived—or died—according to whether they received the "wonder drug of 1943."[19]

The discovery and development of penicillin, aptly described by Gladys Hobby, John Sheehan, Gwyn MacFarlane, and others are familiar to historians of medicine. Limited production created a scarcity of the drug during the Second World War. Although some researchers and pharmaceutical firms had expressed passing interest in penicillin's antibacterial properties, few studies were carried out. Neither Alexander Fleming nor other investigators showed much interest in penicillin. Fleming devoted his attention instead to other projects. According to Milton Wainwright and Harold T. Swan in a 1986 *Medical History* article, Drs. C. G. Paine and A.

Dickson Wright of Britain were among the few physicians who had used topical penicillin as early as 1930.[20]

American and British investigators began by 1940 to investigate the clinical promise of penicillin. Howard Florey in the spring of that year demonstrated the effectiveness of penicillin in the treatment of laboratory animals infected with streptococci, staphylococci, and clostridia; by fall clinicians at Columbia-Presbyterian Medical Center in New York had administered penicillin to a patient with bacterial endocarditis. Although the patient succumbed to this malady, investigators had further demonstrated the clinical potential of penicillin.[21]

As interest in the drug grew, U.S. Department of Agriculture researchers in Peoria, Illinois addressed problems of supplying investigators with sufficient penicillin for clinical trials. Although Squibb had considered the possibility of mass production during the 1930s, the company determined that penicillin research was neither profitable nor practical. Hopes for the development of mass production technology, however, lay in the USDA's biochemists and engineers. The British, whom Florey first approached about producing penicillin for clinical trials on a large scale, had shown relatively little interest in producing the drug. Mass production, British pharmaceutical manufacturers believed, would prove laborious and wasteful—too a great a chance to take on an untested substance. Moreover, subsequent development of synthetic penicillin might render worthless any substantial investments in fermentation technology. In addition, the war effort had placed too great a burden on the British chemical industry. As the *Luftwaffe* pummeled the home island, the British government gave far greater priority to munitions production.[22]

Low penicillin production also slowed American clinical research. However, the vigorous lobbying of top American officials by researchers Howard Florey and Norman Heatley in the summer of 1941 provided the important push that the project needed. By early 1943, the Committee on Medical Research (CMR) Chairman A. N. Richards had convinced leading American drug companies to consider support of penicillin research, and many rushed to provide penicillin for wounded troops.[23]

The entrance of Merck, Squibb, and other pharmaceutical manufacturers into the penicillin effort provided the industrial base for making the drug, but the problem of mass production remained. At first, penicillin was produced by surface culture; however, this method proved painfully slow and inefficient. Corn steep liquor provided a successful alternative, growing the penicillin mold not on the culture's surface but within the medium itself. Once researchers perfected this method and mass production facilities were constructed, American penicillin production increased markedly. Between January and December 1943, Merck alone expanded its penicillin output ninety-fold.[24]

Despite these increases, severe home-front shortages persisted late into the war. Although the manufacturers could provide adequate supplies of the drug for military patients, penicillin remained an extremely scarce home front commodity. Production levels could not meet both the civilian and military demands for the drug. Until sufficient penicillin became available for both civilians and servicemen, however, policy makers required a plan to provide at least *some* of the life-saving drug to the home front.[25]

Bureaucratic administration lay at the heart of the program of wartime penicillin rationing. This type of organization utilizes individuals who enforce official regulations that govern its operation, sociologist Max Weber had argued. Persons who work within a bureaucratic system exercise their authority on the basis of education and expertise, objectively and efficiently executing their duties. Clearly defined guidelines or criteria, which help to minimize subjective considerations, permit a person to exercise authority with detached precision. The "objective discharge" of responsibilities, Weber also had theorized, occurs "without regard for persons," and it eliminates from "official business love, hatred, and all purely personal, irrational, and emotional elements which escape calculation." Legal scholar John T. Noonan, Jr., remarked also that adherence to rules also permits authority figures to depersonalize judgments so that they become merely "players of roles." "Masks," both their own shrouds of authority and those which they apply to persons subject to their authority, cloak "individual human beings so their humanity is hidden and disavowed," Noonan added. Professionals such as judges or physicians may "mask" themselves as the authority structure itself. Their actions then reflect the values of the system rather than their own.[26]

Both the Chairman of the COC and the Director of the Office of Civilian Penicillin Distribution relied upon bureaucratic techniques to distribute penicillin to civilians. The precise language of their policy permitted them (and all who used the drug) to decide who received—and did not receive—penicillin. The criteria for rationing permitted the maintenance of an efficient distribution system as well as objectivity on the part of physicians who determined a patient's eligibility for the drug. The decision on whether or not to provide penicillin for civilian cases represented just another dimension of their wartime responsibilities. Official policy, not personal considerations, remained the only criterion for the release of penicillin to a patient. The depersonalization of actions permitted physicians to exercise their authority while remaining emotionally detached from the harsh reality of their task. They knew the Committee expected them to refuse penicillin to all patients who did not meet specific clinical guidelines.[27]

This triage model had first been used effectively during the Napoleonic Wars in an attempt to deal with large numbers of casualties in an efficient manner. The most serious cases, one of Napoleon Bonaparte's surgeons noted, rated treatment priority *"entirely without regard to rank or distinction."* The less severely injured received treatment only after more serious cases had been attended. Medical need alone dictated the order in which surgeons tended the wounded.[28]

The COC followed a similar triage system that selected civilian cases according to the likelihood of recovery as well as the importance of the disease to the war effort. In the case of military patients, treatment decisions were made in the interest of returning soldiers as quickly as possible to active duty. During the North African campaign, for example, it was common to grant treatment priority to gonorrhea victims because they stood the greatest chance of returning to the field in as short a time as possible, a decision which further suggests the bureaucratic tone of penicillin rationing decisions. Policy makers were far less worried about any moral issues that were involved and far more concerned about the most equitable and efficient rationing of the drug. Although the COC concerned itself primarily with civilian cases, its treatment guidelines mirrored those used in military field hospitals: cases that penicillin could treat effectively and were of military interest received the drug. Neither sex, political influence, age, or any other subjective criteria influenced rationing decisions. Even when the OCPD accepted rationing responsibilities of penicillin in 1944, private physicians were expected to use the drug only on cases that would respond to it. On an administrative level, the bureaucratic policy addressed distributional issues of rationing. On a medical-scientific level, bureaucracy underpinned the "cooperative clinical guidelines" described by Harry Marks.[29]

The COC provided an ideal forum for making rationing decisions. First, each member of the Committee held respected credentials in the field of infectious diseases. Second, the analysis of data on which the COC determined distribution was the primary purpose of the Committee. Bioethicist Marc D. Basson noted that this decision-making process "can be more rational because as a small committee of experts they are isolated from the waves of emotionality and fads that sweep through the general populace periodically." Personal detachment from committee decisions is also of vital importance. It goes without saying that no committee member (or friend or family member) should be a candidate for a particular scarce medical resource. Basson concluded, "Human lives are too important for political games, and the allocation decision would be better left to a committee of experts with the time to gather and assimilate information and the disinterest which permits rational decision making."[30]

Such an attempt at objective adherence to clinical protocol had not always been the case. When Frederick Banting and Charles Best introduced insulin shortly after the First World War, frantic requests for the substance quickly flooded into their Toronto laboratory. One Johns Hopkins pediatrician, for example, stressed that he had "really heart-breaking cases" that desperately needed treatment. Could the Toronto researchers provide any of the life-saving insulin? petitioners begged. "Diabetics," Michael Bliss wrote in *The Discovery of Insulin*, "were literally camping at the doors of the lab trying to get insulin." The extremely short supply of the drug, however, limited the number of cases that Banting could treat. The scarcity of insulin, combined with the public clamor for the drug, forced the Toronto investigators to formulate some type of rationing policy.[31]

Unlike Chester Keefer and the COC, Banting relied upon subjective criteria in his selection of patients, yielding to the weight of political influence and personal considerations. Banting, for example, treated his former medical school classmate, the son of the vice president of Kodak, and the daughter of Secretary of State Charles Evans Hughes. At the same time, he denied other pleas for the drug. On another occasion, he discontinued therapy for five cases so he could treat an elderly patient with a gangrenous leg.[32]

One of Banting's colleagues recalled that he was nearly distraught over the acute shortage of insulin—perhaps because he refused to distance himself from the rationing process. He had great difficulty in deciding to treat one patient but not another. The sober-minded Keefer, on the other hand, shielded himself by following his policy (with only one exception) to the letter. He expected all under his authority to follow his example. Banting's background, however, was in surgery not clinical medicine. Moreover, the insulin studies were carried out a decade prior to the heyday of cooperative clinical investigation. Keefer, who achieved professional prominence a decade or so later, avoided the pitfalls that plagued the insulin researchers.[33]

The bureaucratic policy that guided penicillin rationing meshed easily with the "search for order" that had reached its height during the Roosevelt years. Progressive reformers had hoped that bureaucratic organization would create "a paradise of new-middle class rationality" as budding professionals attempted to rectify societal ills from child labor to corrupt urban political machines. During the First World War, wartime agencies such as the War Industries Board, Fuel Administration, and Committee on Public Information attempted to bring administrative efficiency to the home front effort. During the Great Depression, the federal government continued this trend by placing experts, particularly those in academe, in positions to address the nation's numerous economic and social problems.[34]

The United States' entrance into the Second World War, however, tested the boundaries of "big government." Expanding beyond New Deal limits, the enlarged wartime administration used experts to direct successfully the American military effort. As part of the mobilization, agencies such as the War Production Board controlled the rationing of many war materials; the Office of War Information informed American civilians of news at home and on the front; and the Office of Scientific Research and Development administered wartime scientific and medical research. Each office held responsibility for directing a specific aspect of war effort.[35]

Penicillin rationing at its most basic level differed little from government control of other scarce commodities, and by early 1943 the United States had created over a dozen major rationing programs. Wartime administrators by 1943 oversaw the rationing of sugar, gasoline, and other items; yet, want of these consumer goods usually meant little more than inconvenience for most Americans. A housewife might not have have enough butter and sugar to bake a cake, or a family might postpone Sunday drives for the duration. If a patient were unable to get penicillin, however, he or she might face death rather than mere inconvenience. This issue cast penicillin rationing in a far more serious light.[36]

The professional authority of the academic medical elites appointed to the COC or its team of accredited investigators found a welcome place within wartime bureaucracy. Physicians represented the most logical choice for the distribution of penicillin. Not only could they use their skills to determine a patient's illness, their diagnosis and prognosis provided a guide by which to decide whether the patient qualified for penicillin treatment. The professional status of physicians permitted them to act as "gatekeepers" to the drug. Given the sociopolitical climate of the Roosevelt years and the goals of the penicillin investigative program, the COC distributed the drug in an equitable and efficient manner. Alternative rationing methods, such as random selection of cases, might well have adversely affected the war effort and undermined the entire research program.[37]

The bureaucratic rationing of penicillin at the hands of "managerial elites" did more than streamline the distribution of the drug. The use of impartial clinical criteria was an attempt to insure that all qualified patients received penicillin (as long as sufficient supplies of the drug remained available). As historian William Nelson noted, late nineteenth century reformers had hoped that bureaucracy would provide all persons, without regard to position or influence, equal access to governmental goods and services. He concluded that late nineteenth century reformers "strove to prevent centralization and concentration of power and to institutionalize pluralism." Bureaucratic administration, which had reached its height in the United States by the dawn of the Second World War, sought to protect the rights of all citizens.[38]

The method of penicillin rationing may have also reflected the legal climate of the Roosevelt era. Given the emphasis placed upon the equal protection and due process clauses of the Fifth and Fourteenth Amendments, the use of bureaucracy reflected attempts to insulate the COC's decisions both from charges of inequity and abridgment of due process. The Legal Division of the Office of Scientific Research and Development, for example, counseled the Committee on Medical Research and COC concerning "legally justifiable" grounds on which investigators might ration penicillin.[39]

The rationing policy of the Committee on Chemotherapy (unlike that of Banting) withstood most political, professional, and popular criticism. Attempts by senators, congressmen, and even the Secretary of State, to obtain the drug for a favored constituent proved of little use. Unless the patient had an illness against which penicillin had proven effective, the COC denied treatment. Only in extraordinary cases (in which physicians obtained the drug without the knowledge of the committee chairman) did political influence have any effect upon rationing policy. Despite the flaws in the "distributional formula" of the Office of Civilian Penicillin Distribution, its advisory board attempted to provide access to penicillin in as equitable and objective a manner as possible. As James Jones described in *Bad Blood*, however, such an uncompromising commitment to the bureaucratic process had the potential to transform clinical investigation into a macabre experiment.[40]

Several individuals questioned the authority of the COC. Committee policy, some argued, had stifled promising research avenues, while others complained that Keefer was a coldhearted bureaucrat. The deaths of several highly publicized patients bolstered Chester Keefer's unsavory public image. Conflicting media reports also resulted in the immeasurable heartache and disappointment of those who were unable to obtain treatment with the drug; incorrect news stories bred confusion over the rationing policy of the COC.[41]

Some writers on the wartime treatment of subacute bacterial endocarditis (SBE), for example, have praised those physicians who circumvented the guidelines of the COC. Paul De Kruif noted in 1949 that "some obscure Brooklyn boys had solved this deadliest of all microbic mysteries and had succeeded where medical powers of the National Research Council had failed." The NRC's Committee on Chemotherapy, manned by individuals "within the scientific orbit of the Harvard-Yale-Columbia-Cornell-Johns Hopkins medical axis," refused until 1944 to release penicillin for the treatment of SBE. Throughout, De Kruif's description emphasized the snobbish insensitivity of the "B.C.M. (Big Committee Man)"—Chester Keefer, COC chairman and "the National Research Council's arbiter of who got penicillin and who did not." Advocates of the treatment of SBE, Jack Smith of Pfizer Pharmaceuticals and Dr. Leo Loewe of Brooklyn Jewish Hospital, appear in De Kruif's account as beneficent souls at war with intransigent wartime bureaucrats and *streptococcus viridans* alike.[42]

The most recent discussion of the treatment of wartime SBE appeared in Gladys Hobby's *Penicillin: Meeting the Challenge*. The author argues that the treatment of subacute bacterial endocarditis "came from the humanitarian instincts of a few—perhaps ten or a dozen—persons who were simply concerned for those afflicted with the disease." Hobby retells the heroic efforts of Leo Loewe, Ward MacNeal, M.H. Dawson (with whom she worked closely on the penicillin research), and Pfizer Pharmaceuticals. The perspective of Keefer and the COC, however, receives scant attention in this regard. Hobby notes only that Chester Keefer, pleased that treatment of SBE had finally proven successful in 1944, "admitted [to] the value of penicillin in . . . subacute bacterial endocarditis." By that time, however, increased production of the drug permitted investigators to include SBE in their research.[43]

While some persons objected to penicillin rationing policy, others protested the tight-lipped attitude of the COC and CMR concerning news releases on penicillin. Beginning with the treatment of the Coconut Grove Fire victims in late 1942, information leaks about penicillin sparked public excitement over the drug. By the summer of 1943, the "miracle drug" that the COC and CMR hoped to keep from public knowledge had become a major news item.[44]

The desire of the Office of War Information (OWI) to publicize news of penicillin hindered the efficient rationing of the drug. Chester Keefer and A. N. Richards, the Chairman of the Committee on Medical Research, stressed that news reports had increased the number of civilian requests for the drug and threatened the security of penicillin production techniques. The OWI, however, believed it had a responsibility to keep Americans abreast of wartime news. The agency's director, Elmer Davis, summed up the OWI's position: "Thanks to . . . the endeavor of totalitarian governments to suppress all news and all opinion except what they choose to give out, the truth itself has become a more powerful weapon than ever before." Well-informed Americans, the agency found, were more likely to believe that rationing was "being handled properly," a full seventeen percent more in the public opinion polls. Why, then, shouldn't the government publicize the penicillin effort as completely as possible? Keefer and Richards answered that publicity about the drug simply created a "panic" which the COC could not satisfy at that time.[45]

Independent journalists refused to accept the authority of the OWI—much less that of the COC and CMR—to control publicity about penicillin, and many continued to print stories about the drug. Much to the aggravation of Keefer and Richards, confusing reports led ill civilians to believe that political figures, high-ranking military personnel, or public officials could help laypersons obtain penicillin. As the miracle cures of the "wonder drug of 1943" filled the American press, public pressure intensified to ration more of the drug to civilians—deserving or not.[46]

The glowing reports of penicillin's miracle cures in both popular and professional publications influenced postwar American society. The added effect of clever wartime advertisement, influencing both the lay and professional public, increased the overprescription of antibiotics. The experience of wartime penicillin distribution had little immediate effect on its judicious postwar use, for numerous observers believed that medicine had reached its "golden age." Practitioners for several decades after the war ignored the clinical precision recommended by the COC as the array of antibiotics increased.[47]

With the growth of physicians' ability to intervene surgically and medically, whether through organ transplantation or drug therapy, the question of distributing the scarce supply of penicillin has become pale by comparison. The increasing complexity of distributing scarce supplies was becoming apparent even by 1946 as the rationing of streptomycin faced investigators. But without the wartime emergency, selection of patients and maintenance of clinical protocol was a more difficult issue than penicillin rationing had been. Over the past four decades, issues of equitable access to a potentially life-saving drug or technology have continued to face the medical profession. Rationing of medical resources, David Mechanic noted in the late 1970s, has become a harsh reality of modern health care. "Medical care," he wrote, "*is rationed* whether we like it or not, and we would do well to direct attention to the way such rationing can be applied to promote fairness, professional excellence, and the best use of our financial and social resources."[48]

The penicillin and streptomycin rationing of the 1940s has become the AZT, dialysis machine, and donor organ rationing of the late twentieth century. Wartime penicillin, however, provides an excellent case study of the equitable and efficient distribution of a scarce medical resource. Here is that story.[49]

Notes

1. Mary Ann Baily, " 'Rationing' and American Health Policy," *Journal of Health Politics, Policy and Law* 9 (Fall 1984): 489-501.

2. *Ibid.*

3. *Ibid.*

4. Graham Greene, *The Third Man and The Fallen Idol* (New York, 1981).

5. See for example, Victor R. Fuchs, *Who Shall Live? Health, Economics, and Social Choice* (New York, 1974).

6. See for example, Bill Trent, "Is Media Hype Necessary for Organ Transplants?" *Canadian Medical Association Journal* 130 (15 March 1984): 774-780; Claudia Wallis, "Of Television and Transplants," *Time* (23 June 1986): 68.

7. Wallis, "Of Television and Transplants," 68.

8. *Ibid.*

9. Robert H. Blank, *Rationing Medicine* (New York, 1988), 98-99.

10. "Mother Sued Over Payment for Son's Liver Transplants," *New York Times*, 11 November 1984, sec. A, p. 24; "Fund Is Established for Girl with Five Transplanted Organs," *New York Times*, 29 December 1987, p. 11.

11. J.B., "Organs for Sale: From Marketplace to Jungle," *Hastings Center Report* 16 (February 1986): 3-4; George J. Annas, "Life, Liberty, and the Pursuit of Organ Sales," *Hastings Center Report* 14 (February 1984): 22-23; "Organ Transplants: Preference for the Wealthy," *The Lancet* 1 (22 February 1986): 433-434.

12. J.B., "Organs for Sale," *Hastings Center Report* 16 (February 1986): 3-4; Thomas H. Murray, "The Gift of Life Must Always Remain a Gift," *Discover* (March 1986): 90.

13. Felix T. Rapaport, "A Rational Approach to a Common Goal: The Equitable Distribution of Organs for Transplantation," *Journal of the American Medical Association* 257 (12 June 1987): 3118-3119.

14. See for example, Chester Keefer, "Penicillin: A Wartime Accomplishment," in E. C. Andrus, et al. eds., *Advances in Military Medicine Made by American Investigators Working Under the Sponsorship of the Committee on Medical Research*, vol. II, Science in World War II, Office of Scientific Research and Development Series (Boston, 1948), 719-722; Chester S. Keefer to A. N. Richards, 7 September 1943, Committee on Medical Research Files, Record Group 227, National Archives, Washington, D. C. (hereafter cited as CMR, RG 227); Gina Kolata, "Imminent Marketing of AZT Raises Problems," *Science* 235 (20 March 1987): 1462-1463.

15. Keefer, "Penicillin: A Wartime Accomplishment," 719-722.

16. Richard Polenberg, *War and Society: The United States, 1941-1945* (New York, 1972), 4; Barry D. Karl, *The Uneasy State: The United States, 1915-1945* (Chicago, 1984). The historiography on the American home front is enormous. On women, see Maureen Honey, *Creating Rosie the Riveter: Class, Gender, and Propaganda During World War II* (Amherst, Mass., 1984). For a concise discussion of minority relations, see Roger Daniels, *Concentration Camps USA: Japanese Americans and World War II* (New York, 1972) and Neil A. Wynn, *The Afro-American and the Second World War* (New York, 1976).

17. A. Hunter Dupree, *Science in the Federal Government: A History of Policies and Activities to 1940* (New York, 1957), 3, 301-305, 330; Irvin Stewart, *Organizing Scientific Research for War: The Administrative History of the Office of Scientific Research and Development* (Boston, 1948); Daniel Kevles, *The Physicists: The History of a Scientific Community in Modern America* (New York, 1979); see also Alex Roland, "Science and War," *Osiris*, 2d series, 1 (1985): 263-267.

18. The literature on penicillin is enormous. The most recent works include Gladys L. Hobby, *Penicillin: Meeting the Challenge* (New Haven, 1985); Gwyn MacFarlane, *Alexander Fleming: The Man and the Myth* (Cambridge, Mass., 1984); Ronald Hare, "The Scientific Activities of Alexander Fleming Other than the Discovery of Penicillin," *Medical History* 27 (1983): 347-372; John C. Sheehan, *The Enchanted Ring: The Untold Story of Penicillin* (Cambridge, Mass., 1982); John Patrick Swann, "The Search for Penicillin Synthesis during World War II," *British Journal for the History of Science* 16 (July 1983): 154-190; Milton Wainwright and Harold T. Swan, "C.G. Paine and the Earliest Surviving Clinical Records of Penicillin Therapy," *Medical History* 30 (1986): 42-56; and the collection of essays in John Parascandola, ed., *The History of Antibiotics: A Symposium* (Madison, 1980).

19. W.H. Helfand et al., "Wartime Industrial Development of Penicillin in the United States," in Parascandola, ed., *The History of Antibiotics*, 31-32.

20. Milton Wainwright and Harold T. Swan, "C.G. Paine and the Earliest Surviving Clinical Record of Penicillin Therapy," 30 *Medical History* (1986): 42-56.

21. Gladys L. Hobby, *Penicillin: Meeting the Challenge*, 72-73.

22. Helfand et al., "Wartime Industrial Development of Penicillin in the United States," 33-34.

23. *Ibid.*

24. *Ibid.*, 44.

25. "Supply of Penicillin," *American Journal of Public Health* 34 (January 1944): 93.

26. Max Weber, "Bureaucracy," in Oscar Grusky and George A. Miller, eds., *The Sociology of Organizations: Basic Studies* (New York, 1970), 5-18; John T. Noonan, Jr., *Persons and Masks of the Law: Cardozo, Jefferson, and Wythe as Makers of the Masks* (New York, 1976).

27. Noonan, *Persons and Masks of the Law*; Harry M. Marks, "Notes from the Underground," in Russell C. Maulitz and Diana E. Long, eds., *Grand Rounds: One Hundred Years of Internal Medicine* (Philadelphia, 1988), 297-336.

28. Gerald R. Winslow, *Triage and Justice* (Berkeley, 1982).

29. Marks, "Notes from the Underground," 297-336.

30. Marc D. Basson, "Choosing Among Candidates for Scarce Medical Resources," *Journal of Medicine and Philosophy* 4 (1979): 313-333.

31. Michael Bliss, *The Discovery of Insulin* (Chicago, 1982), 134-137.

32. *Ibid.*, 143-160.

33. *Ibid.*, 45-47.

34. Robert H. Wiebe, *The Search for Order: 1877-1920* (New York, 1967), 170; Lewis Auerbach, "Scientists in the New Deal: A Pre-War Episode in the Re-

lations Between Science and Government in the United States," *Minerva* (1965): 457-482; Robert Kargon and Elizabeth Hodes, "Karl Compton, Isaiah Bowman, and the Politics of Science in the Great Depression," *Isis* 76 (September 1985): 301-318; R. G. Tugwell, *The Brains Trust* (New York, 1968); Eliot A. Rosen, *Hoover, Roosevelt, and the Brains Trust: From Depression to New Deal* (New York, 1977).

35. Dupree, *Science in the Federal Government*, 344-368; Karl, *The Uneasy State*, 231. See especially, Polenberg, *War and Society*; Allan M. Winkler, *The Politics of Propaganda: The Office of War Information, 1942-1945* (New Haven, 1978).

36. Richard R. Lingeman, *Don't You Know There's a War On?* (New York, 1976), 234-270; Paul M. O'Leary, "Wartime Rationing and Government Organization," *American Political Science Review* 34 (December 1945): 1089.

37. At the heart of the concept of a physician's professional authority lies the concept of "cultural authority," which a doctor exercises in order to pass judgment on whether a patient is "really sick." See especially, Paul Starr, *The Social Transformation of American Medicine* (New York, 1982), 13-15; Deborah A. Stone, "Physicians as Gatekeepers: Illness Certification as a Rationing Device," *Public Policy* 27 (Spring 1979): 222-254; Edmund D. Pellegrino, "Rationing Health Care: The Ethics of Medical Gatekeeping," *Journal of Contemporary Health Law and Policy* 2 (1986): 23-45; Eliot Freidson, *Professional Powers: A Study of the Institutionalization of Formal Knowledge* (Chicago, 1986); Thomas L. Haskell, "Introduction," in Thomas L. Haskell, ed., *The Authority of Experts: Studies in History and Theory* (Bloomington, Ind., 1984), ix-xviii.

38. William E. Nelson, *The Roots of American Bureaucracy, 1830-1900* (Cambridge, Mass., 1982), 1-7; Kargon and Hodes, "Karl Compton, Isaiah Bowman, and the Politics of Science in the Great Depression."

39. Paul L. Murphy, *The Constitution in Crisis Times, 1918-1969* (New York, 1972); see also James F. Blumstein, "Rationing Medical Resources: A Constitutional, Legal, and Policy Analysis," *Texas Law Review* 59 (November 1981): 1345-1399; E. Tefft Barker to John T. Connor, 3 September 1943, CMR, RG 227.

40. Proposal of the Task Committee on Civilian Penicillin Distribution, 6 April 1944, 1-8, Record Group 179, War Production Board Files, National Archives, Washington, D.C.; James H. Jones, *Bad Blood: The Tuskegee Syphilis Experiment* (New York, 1981), 180.

41. See especially, Chester S. Keefer to M. H. Dawson, 12 June 1943 and Wallace E. Herrell to Chester S. Keefer, 11 August 1943, CMR, RG 227.

42. Paul De Kruif, *Life Among the Doctors* (New York, 1949), 210-245.

43. Hobby, *Penicillin: Meeting the Challenge*, 161, 169.

44. Jerome S. Bruner, "OWI and the American Public," *Public Opinion Quarterly* 7 (Spring 1943): 126; Elmer Davis, "The OWI Has a Job," *Public Opinion Quarterly* 7 (Spring 1943): 8; and Winkler, *The Politics of Propaganda*, 34-35.

45. *Ibid.*

46. Winkler, *The Politics of Propaganda*, 53.

47. Philip N. Jones, Roy S. Bigham, and Phil R. Manning, "Use of Antibiotics in Nonbacterial Respiratory Infections," *Journal of the American Medical Association* 153 (26 September 1953): 264; Henry E. Simmons and Paul D. Stolley, "This Is Medical Progress? Trends and Consequences of Antibiotic Use in the United States," *Journal of the American Medical Association* 227 (4 March 1974): 1023-1028; John C. Burnham, "American Medicine's Golden Age: What Happened to It?" *Science* 215 (19 March 1982): 1474-1479.

48. David Mechanic, "The Growth of Medical Technology and Bureaucracy: Implications for Medical Care," *Milbank Memorial Fund Quarterly* 55 (Winter 1977): 73-75.

49. Tom L. Beauchamp and James F. Childress, *Principles of Biomedical Ethics* (New York, 1979), 188-200; Henry J. Aaron and William B. Schwartz, *The Painful Prescription: Rationing Hospital Care* (Washington, D.C., 1984); Gina Kolata, "Imminent Marketing of AZT Raises Problems," *Science* 235 (20 March 1987): 1462-1463; David Mechanic, "How Should Medical Care Be Rationed?" *American Journal of Medicine* 66 (January 1979): 8-9.

Chapter One

"Medical Preparedness"

When war erupted in Europe in September 1939, the United States closely monitored hostilities between the Allies and Germany. Although the nation remained neutral, Congress soon approved cash-and-carry arms sales and, less than a year later, an unprecedented peacetime draft. As Germany routed British forces at Dunkirk in May 1940, the Army Surgeon General asked the Division of Medical Sciences (DMS) of the National Research Council (NRC) to establish committees to insure "medical preparedness" for war. By 1945, several dozen committees and subcommittees had been created. One of the first, the Committee on Chemotherapeutic and Other Agents (COC), utilized a team of experts who conducted clinical studies on the treatment of infection. Although the early work of the Committee focused primarily on the sulfonamides, by 1943 the attention of the COC had turned to penicillin. Between May 1940 and summer 1943, the Committee became the central force in the clinical evaluation of penicillin and assumed an important—and often controversial—place in wartime bureaucratic administration.[1]

As during the First World War, the armed forces were again seeking the assistance of the NRC and the DMS. The armed forces desperately required a plan for "medical preparedness" in the event that the United States entered the war against the Axis. Given the admirable record of the NRC and DMS twenty years earlier, the military reasoned, these agencies could serve the United States once again.[2]

Speaking at the annual meeting of the DMS in April 1940, Chairman Lewis H. Weed said the war in Europe would generate "new problems of military medicine." He announced that the Division of Medical Sciences remained ready to serve both the armed forces and the government. Acting as liaison between the DMS and the military, Colonel C. C. Hillman and Commander C. S. Stephenson of the navy medical corps listened intently to Weed's discussion of wartime medical problems. The military establishment had thus taken an important step in enlisting the assistance of American medical researchers.[3]

When Surgeon General James Magee contacted Weed on May 14, 1940, he stressed that "the disturbed international situation" had created several areas of concern for the army. Magee said he understood that Weed frequently visited Washington and had expressed his desire to discuss cooperative projects with the DMS. Weed agreed, and two days later the surgeon general's office arranged a meeting for the seventeenth with Weed, Colonel Hillman and Colonel J. S. Simmons.[4]

Their conference created the first two of over a dozen wartime committees of the Division of Medical Sciences, one to study drugs such as the sulfonamides in the treatment of battle wounds (the COC), the other to conduct research on blood transfusions. Both reflected central medical concerns from the First World War. While the COC investigated effective treatment of infections, the Committee on Transfusions studied problems of shock and blood replacement. Eager to implement their work, Colonel Hillman informed Weed on May 21 that he believed that a close relationship should be forged as soon as possible between the Division of Medical Sciences and the armed forces. He emphasized that his office also welcomed the assistance of the Public Health Service and the navy.[5]

The army respected the abilities of the Division of Medical Sciences, for the agency had served the military admirably during the First World War. "With the exception of its futile efforts to check the influenza epidemic, the record of medicine in the war was so outstanding that it introduced a new era of warfare in which the diseases that had once ravaged armies and civilians alike were kept under control," historian of science A. Hunter Dupree noted.[6]

"Even as late as the Spanish-American War, when the bacteria responsible for many infections had been discovered," one contemporary observer added, "certain diseases, particularly typhoid fever, caused crippling epidemics, thus reflecting the inadequate state of contemporary knowledge about their epidemiology and prevention." Despite the shining record of military medicine during the First World War, COC member John Lockwood was to note in spring 1942, there remained room for improvement. Fifty-eight thousand soldiers had died from disease alone, he wrote. By 1918, mortality had reached twenty-seven per thousand soldiers in the field.[7]

Weed, acting on the authority of the Chairman of the National Research Council, on May 21, 1940 appointed Perrin H. Long, Francis G. Blake, John S. Lockwood, John Mahoney, and E. K. Marshall, Jr., to the COC. The army surgeon general, he explained, had asked him to organize a team of researchers to advise the military concerning "the prophylactic and curative use of chemotherapeutic and other agents." It was an important consideration, Harry Marks has noted, that the perspectives of a number of experienced investigators be utilized to insure objective clinical research. Large numbers of patients, he added, could offset the possibility of spontaneous recoveries. Of even greater importance, however, was the selection of clinicians who could be relied upon to conduct their research according to a predetermined investigative protocol.[8]

Each of the Committee appointees, selected at the conference between Weed, Hillman, and Simmons, was expert in the field of infectious diseases and their treatment, but perhaps none was as well known as its original Chairman, Perrin Long. Such a highly respected researcher and able administrator, the Division of Medical Sciences reasoned, could manage the work of the Committee most efficiently. By the late 1930s, Long had acquired an outstanding reputation. After receiving his medical degree from the University of Michigan in 1924, Long accepted a one-year fellowship at Boston's Thorndike Laboratory and spent two more years under the tutelage of the renowned Francis Peabody. In 1927, after several months at the Hygienic Institute in Freiburg, Germany, Long joined the staff of the Rockefeller Institute. Two years later, he became Director of the Biological Division of the Osler Clinic at Johns Hopkins.[9]

Throughout the 1930s, he and his colleagues published studies on the common cold, influenza, and whooping cough. In 1939, Long produced *The Clinical and Experimental Use of Sulfanilamide, Sulfapyridine and Allied Compounds*, a pioneering study coauthored with Eleanor Bliss. (Long's professional reputation, one colleague recalled, was to earn him a place among a group of experts selected to advise the military about the treatment of Pearl Harbor casualties.)[10]

At the first meeting of the COC on May 28, 1940, Division of Medical Sciences Chairman Weed reiterated that the escalating situation in Europe and the Far East required the immediate organization of expert investigators to be "at the disposal of the Government at all times." No one could predict, he warned, when the United States might be drawn into war.[11] Following Weed's introductory remarks, Committee Chairman Perrin Long invited the military representatives, James Magee and C. S. Stephenson, to present their requirements concerning the treatment of battlefield wounds and infections.[12]

Magee and Stephenson outlined six specific areas of military concern for the COC: 1) efficacy of antitoxins in wounds infected with *Clostridium welchii* and other anaerobic organisms common in cases of gas gangrene; 2) physiological and therapeutic effects of topical "chemotherapeutic agents" (such as sulfanilamide) in septic war wounds; 3) "evaluation and comparison" of local antiseptic agents; 4) use of splinting in traumatic injuries; 5) evaluation of the relative effectiveness of oral and local chemotherapeutic prophylaxis; and 6) "investigation into the present bacteriology of mixed infections." To assist with research in these areas, the Committee formed subcommittees dealing with areas that ranged from surgical infections to tropical diseases. By 1941, the overall number of committees and subcommittees operating under the Division of Medical Sciences had reached nearly forty.[13]

The COC focused its initial attention upon the sulfonamides. The first of these, sulfanilamide, had proven particularly effective in the treatment of Group A hemolytic streptococcal, gonococcal, and meningococcal illnesses.[14] Prior to the introduction of the sulfa drugs, streptococcal infections, for example, had remained largely resistant to treatment. A typical medical textbook, published just prior to the introduction of the sulfonamides, noted that the physician could do little to limit "the growth activities of the streptococcus inside the human body." Treatment, therefore, consisted of keeping "the infected area clean and, if possible drained." Unchecked streptococcal infections, the text continued, proved especially debilitating.[15]

Despite the usefulness of the sulfonamides against a number of bacterial infections, researchers sought additional therapeutic agents. The sulfa drugs, for example, had demonstrated little effect on staphylococcal organisms. The Committee in October 1940, thus, gave initial consideration to penicillin. Probably referring to Howard Florey's research published several months earlier in the *British Medical Journal*, Long recommended that the COC pursue investigation of the drug. As soon as he obtained a sample of the substance, Long promised to provide additional details to the Committee. Scarcity of the drug, because of low production and the limited funding for the Division of Medical Sciences, prevented large-scale clinical investigation of penicillin at that time.[16] Prior to the perfection of deep fermentation methods, critical in providing adequate penicillin during the latter half of the war, researchers laboriously produced penicillin mold on surface cultures in one-liter glass flasks or flat pans containing a growth medium.[17]

Other American researchers had also initiated early studies of penicillin in 1940. Encouraged by the work of Florey and his associates, Martin Henry Dawson and his colleagues at the College of Physicians and Surgeons, Columbia University, corroborated the British research in September 1940. Within a month, Dawson had administered the drug to two patients. Although the small amount of penicillin had not elicited a therapeutic response, the drug had completely inhibited the growth of the infecting organisms, Group A beta-hemolytic streptococci.[18]

Other studies confirmed the antibacterial properties of penicillin. In May 1941, Dawson and his colleagues reported to the American Society for Clinical Investigation that penicillin had demonstrated remarkable effectiveness both *in vivo* and *in vitro*. "It is apparently not inhibited by blood and serum, nor by pus and other substances which are known to inhibit the sulfonamides," Dawson commented. The drug also appeared relatively nontoxic. The report concluded on a hopeful note: "Penicillin probably represents a new class of chemotherapeutic agents which may prove as useful or even more useful than the sulfonamides."[19]

At the December 1941 meeting of the American Society of Bacteriologists, Gladys Hobby, one of Dawson's coworkers, confirmed Dawson's findings. She reported that penicillin had proven highly effective against a broad spectrum of bacteria, and it compared favorably with the sulfa drugs. With the drug's great potential established, the clinical research and development of mass production still lay ahead.[20]

The Committee on Medical Research played a critical role in supporting the wartime penicillin program. Created under the Office of Scientific Research and Development in June 1941, the agency investigated "medical problems related to national defense" and coordinated the efforts of American medical and scientific researchers. Through funding by the Office of Emergency Management, the Committee contracted individual researchers, institutions, the National Academy of Sciences, National Research Council, and other groups to pursue war-related research. The assistance of these groups, the Committee on Medical Research hoped, would permit the most efficient and comprehensive approach to the administration of wartime research.[21]

The Committee on Medical Research in January 1942 gave the COC the responsibility for the clinical evaluation of penicillin. CMR Chairman A. N. Richards assured Perrin Long that, despite production problems, he could expect to have enough of the drug for limited clinical trials. At its next meeting on February 4, 1942, the Committee concluded that, since the sulfonamides had proven ineffective against staphylococcal infections—all too common in field hospitals—this condition "offered the best chance for evaluating the therapeutic effects of [penicillin]." As supplies of the drug increased, the COC concluded that a team of researchers to include Champ Lyons, Chester Keefer, Francis Blake, Martin Henry Dawson, and Wesley Spink should initiate these studies. Each was respected in the clinical investigation of infectious diseases, and the COC believed they could produce useful research data in the shortest possible time.[22]

By the summer of 1942, studies by these investigators had shown that penicillin could inhibit the growth of *staphylococci*. These promising results prompted the COC and CMR to enlarge their research program. As a result, the Committee on Chemotherapy added pneumococcal meningitis and empyema, sulfonamide-resistant puerperal infections, and (for a short time) subacute bacterial endocarditis to its investigative agenda. To organize forthcoming reports, the Committee appointed Dr. Chester S. Keefer of its Subcommittee on Infectious Diseases. Keefer served at the time as information coordinator, responsible for collection and interpretation of clinical data on penicillin. During this period, Keefer became more closely involved in the administrative aspect of the COC—experience that proved extremely useful when he assumed the chairmanship of the Committee later that year.[23]

The resignation of Chairman Perrin Long in late August 1942 opened a new phase in the history of the Committee. DMS Chairman Lewis Weed hoped to replace Long with an individual who combined strong administrative skills and outstanding clinical qualifications. On September 1, 1942, less than a week after Long had formally left the Committee, Weed offered the chairmanship of the COC to Chester Keefer. "My dear Doctor Keefer," he wrote, "Dr. Perrin H. Long has resigned chairmanship of the Committee on Chemotherapeutic and Other Agents . . . in order to accept a commission in the Army of the United States." Weed added, "It is the general consensus that the Committee will function better under your chairmanship than that of any other individual." Speaking for the Division of Medical Sciences, Weed said he hoped that Keefer would agree to head the COC; he accepted the position several days later.[24]

Chester Keefer was an ideal choice. Not only did he enjoy an outstanding professional reputation in clinical investigation, he had gained administrative experience as Wade Professor of Medicine and Chairman at Boston University School of Medicine, Director of the Evans Department of Clinical Research and Preventive Medicine, and Physician-in-Chief of the University Hospital. He had also served as information coordinator for the COC, as a member of the Subcommittee on Infectious Diseases, and as liaison to the Committee on Medical Research. After graduating from Johns Hopkins Medical School in 1922, Keefer remained there as a resident house officer until 1926; he gained additional clinical experience at the University of Chicago and the Peking Union Medical College in China. In 1930, Keefer accepted positions as Assistant Professor of Medicine at Harvard and researcher at the Thorndike Laboratory of Boston City Hospital. By 1940, he had assumed his prestigious position at Boston University School of Medicine. Keefer also published on a variety of topics including hemolytic streptococcal diseases and gonococcal arthritis. Between 1923, the year Keefer's first article appeared, and 1940, he produced an average of eight publications annually.[25]

Weed on September 2 also appointed W. Barry Wood, Jr., to the Committee. After graduating from Johns Hopkins Medical School in 1936, he remained there for several years, accepting a research fellowship in bacteriology at Harvard Medical School in 1939. From 1940 until 1942, Wood taught at Hopkins until Washington University in St. Louis offered him a professorship in medicine and the post of physician-in-chief at its teaching facility, Barnes Hospital. With the addition of Wood, the Committee's membership formally consisted of Chairman Chester S. Keefer, Francis G. Blake, John S. Lockwood, E. K. Marshall, Jr., and Wood.[26]

During the fall of 1942, penicillin remained at the top of the COC's agenda, and in mid-October Keefer offered CMR Chairman Richards his assessment of penicillin research. The "evidence" of the "accredited investigators," expert researchers specifically chosen to assist the clinical investigation of penicillin, had confirmed its therapeutic value. The drug had proven especially effective against staphylococcal infections and hemolytic streptococcal infections with bacteremia, chronic osteomyelitis, and chronic empyema. It had shown little clinical effect, however, against subacute bacterial endocarditis. Surveying the evidence, Keefer recommended that future studies concentrate on acute and chronic staphylococcal infections as well as sulfonamide-resistant gram positive infections.[27]

Staphylococcal infections could prove especially serious. Although treatment of localized staphylococcal infections were sometimes "successful," a 1934 textbook advised, therapy remained "largely unsuccessful with regard to the treatment of severe general infection. This does not mean that all cases of severe staphylococcal bacteriemia [sic] are fatal," the author added, "but means that there is no method of treatment which brings about recovery with any degree of certainty." Most cases required surgery, since vaccines remained "inert," and sera had not yet been developed "to a point of assured usefulness." The text concluded grimly that successful "recovery depends on the native resources of the patient." These infections, resistant to the sulfonamides, typically had a mortality rate of over seventy-five percent.[28]

Yet clinicians were growing more convinced of penicillin's potential. A Massachusetts General Hospital study of infections at the end of 1942 provided further evidence of penicillin's effectiveness. Champ Lyons, working under a Committee on Medical Research contract in conjunction with the COC, treated over 170 patients with the drug, nearly a quarter of whom were victims of Boston's Coconut Grove Fire in late 1942. He concluded that the results of penicillin therapy in these cases were extremely "impressive."[29]

Extended clinical trials, however, depended upon adequate supplies of penicillin. Although researchers at the Northern Regional Research Laboratory at Peoria, Illinois, were attempting to overcome production difficulties, commercial producers still expressed concern about the promotion, manufacture, and distributional costs of the drug. Reflecting upon the reticence of American drug companies to apply all their energies to the development of penicillin, Chester Keefer wryly observed that "there is a limit to which any firm can ... venture capital at present without a reasonable chance of return."[30] American pharmaceutical manufacturers resisted large-scale production of penicillin, Gladys Hobby noted, because they feared "that the penicillin-producing mold would contaminate other products on which they depended for sales and revenues," or the new drug might prove too toxic when administered in clinical trials.[31]

The reluctance of pharmaceutical companies to manufacture penicillin restricted the availability of the drug for military personnel and civilians alike. Clinical results, Keefer insisted, remained too sketchy for extensive field application. In January 1943, when the Army tried to obtain the drug from Merck Pharmaceuticals for an officer serving in the Middle East, Keefer stressed that penicillin remained experimental and in extremely short supply. Only the Committee on Medical Research, he added, would release penicillin for field use through the surgeon general.[32]

The military had employed relatively little penicillin up to that time, so the sulfonamides had served as a standard treatment. Not only were these drugs generally available, they were ideal for battlefield use. Soldiers could easily carry—and administer—sulfanilamide powder and sulfadiazine tablets. So important were these drugs that, by early 1942 the Office of the Surgeon General made sulfanilamide standard issue to all troops stationed in a war zone.[33]

The sulfonamides exhibited several problems, however. Not only were they ineffective against staphylococcal infections, they caused "confusion or other mental disturbances," inhibited motor skills, and caused vomiting and nausea in nearly twelve percent of patients. Nearly seven percent of the cases treated with sulfadiazine, considered a more easily tolerated drug, also suffered these symptoms. One wartime investigator recalled, "Penicillin was to make a dramatic entrance into the management of infections and sepsis during World War II. By 1942 the general use of the sulfonamides in medical practice would gradually abate."[34]

The toxicity and limitations of the sulfonamides, combined with the growing body of promising data on penicillin, suggested the great potential of the new drug. Keefer told Richards in late March 1943 that he had given particular consideration to the use of penicillin in the armed forces. The COC Chairman was eager to extend investigations to the military, but to achieve this goal, adequate supplies of the drug were essential: "*We must all push its production as hard as possible* [italics in original]," Keefer stressed.[35]

Keefer based his conclusions on an analysis of "all the reports of wound infections" that had crossed his desk, including data from about two hundred cases that had received penicillin. According to these findings, the sulfonamides had demonstrated particular effectiveness in reducing "the number of *invasive* infections, and the number of deaths." He recommended that "they should be used in all wounded men." However, the effectiveness of these drugs was limited, especially in the treatment of established staphylococcal, clostridial, and streptococcal infections that plagued wounded soldiers.[36]

At the request of Major Frank B. Queen, a medical officer at Bushnell Hospital in Brigham, Utah, Keefer proposed a pilot study to demonstrate the application of penicillin among military casualties. Earlier that month, Queen had informed Keefer of the hospital's two hundred "orthopedic cases many of whom have compound fractures with osteomyelitis and various other complications." The staff, he commented, hoped to use penicillin on patients for whom the sulfa drugs had proven ineffective.[37]

Bushnell Hospital, Keefer believed, provided an ideal opportunity to evaluate penicillin on military casualties. "Arrangements should be made for testing it in these patients in army hospitals," Keefer stressed to Richards. However, he suggested a less direct approach in dealing with the army. "If we put it on the basis of treating patients rather than experimenting with it," Keefer told Richards, "the army will be more receptive." To accomplish this, the COC chairman suggested sending an experienced clinical investigator to military hospitals in order to "get the staff started off in the right direction, and collect observations for use elsewhere." To insure enough penicillin for the project, Keefer continued, Richards should seriously discuss this matter with the nation's leading pharmaceutical manufacturers. Furthermore, he added, Richards needed to secure the approval of the Office of the Surgeon General. It would be improper to initiate military trials without the knowledge of the armed forces. Within a few weeks, Richards and Keefer had received the go-ahead from the surgeon general.[38]

Keefer also convinced his friend (and member of the Committee on Medical Research), A. Baird Hastings, to discuss the program of military trials with "the Chief"—Richards. He suggested that Hastings pound on Richards's desk and stress that "we've got to get penicillin to those returned casualties from the South Pacific suffering from septic war wounds at the Bushnell General Hospital in Brigham, Utah." If Richards agreed, Keefer told Hastings, "tell him Champ Lyons at the MGH [Massachusetts General Hospital] has the know-how and is ready to leave today."[39]

Keefer's letter and Hasting's lobbying simply confirmed what Richards already suspected. After all, the CMR Chairman had been a leading organizer of the penicillin effort by British and American scientists and the American pharmaceutical industry. Richards wrote to Keefer on March 24 that he agreed that penicillin research should be given top priority and that Bushnell Hospital provided an excellent opportunity to study the drug further. Keefer was prepared for the CMR chairman's approval, and he telegrammed in reply, "Lyons willing to go to Utah for study."[40]

Keefer then informed Major Queen, chief of laboratory services at Bushnell, that he had selected Champ Lyons, a member of the Subcommittee on Surgical Infections, to conduct the study. He felt deeply grateful for the opportunity, and he thanked Queen for his "interest in penicillin, and for the facilities which are available for its clinical trials." After reiterating his appreciation to the Hospital's chief of surgery, Colonel Henry Hollenberg, Keefer remarked confidently, "I know that you will find the study of penicillin most fascinating."[41]

When Keefer learned that Champ Lyons had found the Bushnell Project "an extraordinary opportunity . . . to test the usefulness of penicillin," he told Richards, "I have very good news for you." Not only had the Bushnell project commenced smoothly, but "Surgeon General Magee visited the hospital and approved wholeheartedly with the program." The institution had also extended every courtesy to Lyons, providing an entire ward, complete "with individual rooms, an adequate staff, and an excellent laboratory . . . for making adequate bacteriological studies." Keefer added, "Dr. Lyons was most enthusiastic and said that he had a better opportunity to study the cases than he had in Boston."[42]

Lyons's extensive knowledge of bacteriology and surgery and his warm personality impressed the Bushnell staff. Major Queen noted that not only had the study progressed well, but the commanding officer had complimented Lyons's work. The young surgeon had earned the respect of "the entire staff . . . through his active participation in our meetings, his ready willingness to see all of the patients anyone wishes his opinion on, and of course, his sound clinical judgment has been impressive to all," Queen reported to Keefer. The Bushnell physicians were especially fond of Lyons's friendly demeanor, the major continued. Concluding his letter, he remarked, "We are indebted to [you] then for two things: first, for permitting us to have penicillin; and second, for your selection of Dr. Lyons as the man to bring it to us."[43]

Lyons's work at Bushnell clearly demonstrated the military importance of penicillin. On April 22, 1943, he submitted a progress report to Richards, which included the clinical data from nine patients treated between April 5 and April 19. Of those cases, five had been wounded on Guadalcanal in the fall and winter of 1942-1943, one by bomb fragments in Alaska ten months earlier, while the remaining three were civilian patients. Despite their chronic, sulfonamide-resistant infections, some lingering for nearly a year, these patients were effectively treated with penicillin. Lyons's results had so greatly impressed the military that the surgeon general had agreed to "buy the major part of 150,000,000 units [of penicillin] a week for use in clinical investigations in army hospitals." One medical advisor predicted that by mid-September 1943 the army would require nearly five billion units of penicillin each week.[44]

Drug companies eagerly responded to the increased requirement for penicillin. Although only five American companies—Merck, Squibb, Pfizer, Winthrop, and Abbott—were involved in the production of the drug by the summer of 1943, numerous other firms later joined them. Their concerted efforts were instrumental in boosting monthly penicillin supplies from less than a billion units in July 1943 to nearly 130 billion units a year later.[45]

Bushnell Hospital continued to hum with excitement. Judging from the military's reaction to the results of the study, Lyons wrote, "the way is clear for controlled extension of therapy in military hospitals under a liaison agreement with the C.M.R." Since Major Queen planned to continue the Bushnell study, Lyons concluded that his own work at the hospital was complete. By the middle of May the surgeon general had formally asked Lyons to establish wound infection study units at nearly a dozen other facilities. The results of Lyons's work were so striking, Keefer recalled several years later, that they convinced the medical corps of the drug's enormous military importance.[46]

The Bushnell studies represented a turning point in the clinical evaluation of penicillin by the COC. Not only had the army decided to use penicillin, but this decision left accredited investigators with far less of the drug available for civilian patients. To announce this, A. N. Richards sent the Committee on Medical Research's official statement on penicillin to Morris Fishbein, the editor of the *Journal of the American Medical Association* and head of the Division of Medical Sciences' Committee on Information. "It would be advantageous," he told Fishbein, "if it could be published with the least possible delay, particularly in view of the number of articles which are now coming out in the lay press." Fishbein wasted little time, printing Richards's announcement the following week.[47]

In the statement, Richards outlined the general history and use of penicillin, and then presented a far more important message. Unless penicillin production increased, he emphasized, supplies for civilians would become even more scarce. On May 25, Chester Keefer dispatched a similar memorandum to the accredited investigators. Within a week, he announced, they could anticipate a severe reduction in their supply of penicillin. Because the army and navy would receive most of the drug, he advised the investigators "to greatly reduce the number of patients that you propose to treat." Less than two months later, the "Freeze Order" of the War Production Board had reduced the penicillin to the Committee on Chemotherapy to approximately fifteen percent of the total U. S. production of the drug. From July 1943 until December 1943, for example, the amount of penicillin available to civilian patients averaged only around a half billion units per month. The vast majority of the penicillin produced in the United States went for military use.[48]

By the summer of 1943, the COC had played an important role in the army's program of "medical preparedness" and had assumed a critical position in wartime medical research. Foremost, the Committee had conducted studies which demonstrated the effectiveness of penicillin against organisms resistant to the sulfonamides. In doing so, the function of the Committee had unexpectedly changed. Not only had it transcended its original relationship with the Division of Medical Sciences and National Research Council, the success of the Committee's pencillin research had thrust it and its members into the public eye. Chester Keefer was especially affected as popular excitement over the drug increased in 1943 and early 1944 and its home front supplies dwindled. The clamor transformed Chester Keefer, more than any other individual involved in wartime penicillin research, from academic clinician to penicillin "czar," who authorized treatment only of cases that would yield clinical data of use to the war effort.

Notes

1. George B. Darling, "How the National Research Council Streamlined Medical Research for War," in Morris Fishbein, ed., *Doctors at War* (New York, 1945), 366; Sanford V. Larkey, "The National Research Council and Medical Preparedness," *War Medicine* 1 (January 1941): 79; Chester S. Keefer, "Penicillin: A Wartime Accomplishment," in *Advances in Military Medicine Made by American Investigators Working Under the Sponsorship of the Committee on Medical Research*, vol. II, Science in World War II, Office of Scientific Research and Development Series, (Boston, 1948), 719-722; Robert Dallek, *Franklin D. Roosevelt and American Foreign Policy, 1932-1945* (New York, 1979), 530-532.

2. Dupree, *Science in the Federal Government*, 328-330.

3. Larkey, "The National Research Council and Medical Preparedness," 79. In Committees on Military Medicine documents, "Stephenson" is spelled as it is in the text. In *Doctors at War*, edited by Morris Fishbein, it is spelled "Stevenson."

4. James C. Magee to Lewis H. Weed, 14 May 1940; J.F. Sullivan to Dr. [Lewis H.] Weed, 16 May 1940, Committees on Military Medicine Files, Committee on Chemotherapeutic and Other Agents, National Academy of Sciences, Washington, D.C. [hereafter cited as COMM, NAS].

5. C. C. Hillman to Lewis H. Weed, 21 May 1940, COMM, NAS.

6. Dupree, *Science in the Federal Government*, 316.

7. James Stevens Simmons, "Preventive Medicine in the Army," in *Doctors at War* (New York, 1945), 140; John S. Lockwood to A. N. Richards, 6 April 1942, Committee on Medical Research Files, Record Group 227, National Archives, Washington, D.C. [hereafter cited as CMR, RG 227].

8. Lewis H. Weed to Perrin H. Long, Francis Blake, John Lockwood, John Mahoney, and E.K. Marshall, Jr., 21 May 1940; "List suggested after conference with Cols. Hillman and Simmons," n.d., COMM, NAS; Harry M. Marks, "Notes from the Underground: The Social Organization of

Therapeutic Research, 1920-1950," in Diana Long and Russell Maulitz, eds., *Grand Rounds: One Hundred Years of Internal Medicine* (Philadelphia, 1988), 297-336.

9. A. McGehee Harvey, *Science at the Bedside: Clinical Research in American Medicine, 1905-1945* (Baltimore, 1981), 181-182.

10. Robert Austrian, "Perrin Hamilton Long, 1899-1965," *Transactions of the Association of American Physicians* 79 (1966): 60.

11. "Committee on Chemotherapeutic and Other Agents, Minutes of First Meeting, 28 May 1940," 1-2, COMM, NAS.

12. *Ibid.*, 2-3.

13. *Ibid.*, 3-7. *Clostridium welchii* was of particular concern to the armed forces because approximately 75 percent of all gas gangrene cases in the First World War were contaminated with this organism. Hans Zinsser and Stanhope Bayne-Jones, *A Textbook of Bacteriology*, 8th ed., rev. (New York, 1939), 620-625.

14. Wesley W. Spink, *Infectious Diseases: Prevention and Treatment in the Nineteenth and Twentieth Centuries* (Minneapolis, 1978), 83.

15. Ralph A. Kinsella, "The Coccal Diseases," in *Internal Medicine: Its Theory and Practice in Contributions by American Authors*, 2d ed. (Philadelphia, 1934), 124.

16. "Division of Medical Sciences, Committee on Chemotherapeutic and Other Agents, Minutes of the Fourth Meeting, 12 October 1940," 8, COMM, NAS; Gladys L. Hobby, *Penicillin: Meeting the Challenge* (New Haven, 1985), 142.

17. Baxter, *Scientists Against Time*, 343.

18. Hobby, *Penicillin: Meeting the Challenge*, 72.

19. Quoted in *Ibid.*, 73.

20. *Ibid.*, 79.

21. Irvin Stewart, *Organizing Scientific Research for War: The Administrative History of the Office of Scientific Research and Development* (Boston, 1948), 37; W. H. Helfand, et al., "Wartime Industrial Development of Penicillin in

the United States," in John Parascandola, ed., *The History of Antibiotics: A Symposium* (Madison, 1980), 31-56.

22. A.N. Richards to Perrin H. Long, 24 January 1942, CMR, RG 227.

23. "Committee on Chemotherapeutic and Other Agents, Minutes of 13th Meeting, June 16, 1942," 1-4, COMM, NAS; Marks, "Notes from the Underground," in Long and Maulitz, eds., *Grand Rounds*.

24. Stewart, *Organizing Scientific Research for War*, 106; Perrin H. Long to Lewis H. Weed, 27 August 1942; Lewis H. Weed to Chester S. Keefer, 1 September 1942; Chester S. Keefer to Lewis H. Weed, 4 September 1942, COMM, NAS.

25. Harvey, *Science at the Bedside*, 268-269; Robert W. Wilkins, "Chester Scott Keefer: 1897-1972," *Transactions of the Association of American Physicians* 85 (1972): 24-26.

26. Lewis H. Weed to W. Barry Wood, Jr., 2 September 1942; W. Barry Wood, Jr., 5 September 1942, COMM, NAS. "Wood, Dr. W(illiam) Barry, Jr.," in *American Men of Science: A Biographical Directory* (Lancaster, Penn., 1949), 2759. Although initially appointed to the Committee on Chemotherapeutic and Other Agents, John F. Mahoney was no longer listed as a member of the Committee by 1943. He did, however, contribute important research findings on venereal diseases and their treatment with the sulfonamides and penicillin while Director of the Venereal Disease Research Laboratory and a member of the subcommittee on venereal diseases.

27. Chester S. Keefer to A. N. Richards, 13 October 1942, CMR, RG 227; Marks, "Notes from the Underground," in Long and Maulitz, eds., *Grand Rounds* also provides an excellent analysis of the organization of clinical research in the 1930s and 1940s.

28. Kinsella, "The Coccal Diseases," in *Internal Medicine*, 119; Spink, *Infectious Diseases*, 266.

29. Champ Lyons, "Committee on Medical Research of the Office of Scientific Research and Development: Final Report for the 12 Months Ending December 31, 1942," 17 March 1943, CMR, RG 227.

30. Chester S. Keefer to A. N. Richards, 13 October 1942, CMR, RG 227.

31. Hobby, *Penicillin: Meeting the Challenge*, 109-110.

32. E. C. Andrus to A. N. Richards, 21 January 1943, CMR, RG 227.

33. "Committee on Chemotherapeutic and Other Agents, Minutes of 13th Meeting," 16 June 1942, 3, COMM, NAS.

34. *Ibid.*, 2-3; Spink, *Infectious Diseases*, 84-86; see also, Harry F. Dowling, *Fighting Infection: Conquests of the Twentieth Century* (Cambridge, Mass., 1977), 105-124.

35. Hobby, *Penicillin: Meeting the Challenge*, 142; Chester S. Keefer to A. N. Richards, 22 March 1943, CMR, RG 227.

36. Chester S. Keefer to A. N. Richards, 22 March 1943, CMR, RG 227.

37. *Ibid.*

38. *Ibid.*

39. A. B. Hastings, "Chester Scott Keefer, M.D., D. Sc.: Physician and Teacher, Extraordinary," *The Boston Medical Quarterly* 14 (September 1963): 89-90.

40. A. N. Richards to Chester S. Keefer, 24 March 1943, CMR, RG 227; John C. Sheehan, *The Enchanted Ring: The Untold Story of Penicillin* (Cambridge, Mass., 1982), 18-78.

41. Chester S. Keefer to Frank B. Queen, 26 March 1943; Chester S. Keefer to Henry Hollenberg, 26 March 1943, CMR, RG 227.

42. George F. Lull to Commanding Officer, Bushnell General Hospital, 27 March 1943; Champ Lyons to A. N. Richards, 1 April 1943; Chester S. Keefer to A. N. Richards, 5 April 1943, CMR, RG 227.

43. Frank B. Queen to Chester S. Keefer, 8 April 1943, CMR, RG 227.

44. Champ Lyons to A. N. Richards, 22 April 1943; A. N. Richards to Champ Lyons, 29 April 1943; Paul R. Robinson to the Committee on Medical Research, 17 June 1943, CMR, RG 227.

45. Hobby, *Penicillin: Meeting the Challenge*, 171-197.

46. Champ Lyons to A. N. Richards, 11 May 1943; Chester S. Keefer to A. N. Richards, 11 May 1943, CMR, RG 227.

47. A. N. Richards to Morris Fishbein, 14 May 1943, CMR, RG 227; A. N. Richards, "Penicillin: Statement Released by Committee on Medical

Research," *Journal of the American Medical Association* 122 (22 May 1943): 235-236.

48. A. N. Richards, "Penicillin: Statement Released by Committee on Medical Research," 235; Chester S. Keefer, "Memorandum on Penicillin Distribution," 25 May 1943, CMR, RG 227; Hobby, *Penicillin: Meeting the Challenge*, 142-143, 196; Dowling, *Fighting Infection*, 132-134.

Chapter Two

Out of the Ivory Tower

Academic physicians by 1940 had acquired considerable status within the medical profession. University-affiliated medical professors devoted their full attention to teaching and research at the nation's leading research institutes and medical schools. As war threatened, the Roosevelt administration sought their expertise in the same way that it had secured the assistance of academics during the New Deal. Clinical investigators had gained particular professional prestige and authority through their research, through affiliation with leading teaching hospitals, medical schools, and clinics, and through the efforts of the American Society for Clinical Investigation.[1]

The physicians to be appointed to the COC had become by 1940 leading authorities in clinical investigation. Trained in (and later affiliated with) the finest medical schools, teaching hospitals, and research institutes, they produced important work in the field of infectious diseases and continued on to assume prestigious academic posts. Their reputations as clinical investigators made them outstanding choices for the COC. Studying the treatment of wartime infections, Committee members applied their expertise to solve critical problems of military medicine. Although some civilians (both laymen and physicians) objected to the role of the COC in penicillin rationing, the academics of the Committee were best suited for the distribution of the drug. Had the Committee not based penicillin rationing upon objective clinical guidelines, access to the drug might have been based upon criteria such as a patient's social status, political influence, financial assets, or humanitarian motives.[2]

Early twentieth century academic physicians had assumed responsibility for conducting medical research and disseminating their findings to their students. By 1910, the 131 medical schools in the United States employed over six hundred faculty members with full-time salaried positions. Since over a third of the institutions completely lacked salaried instructors, the most prestigious institutions averaged over a half dozen full-time professors each. These individuals, most of whom held full-time faculty positions at prominent eastern institutions, were researchers and teachers—not practitioners. The professors at these institutions felt responsible for the improvement of American medical education.[3]

The efforts of academic physicians yielded professional repute instead of financial reward outside the university setting. One of the Johns Hopkins Medical School faculty members commented that medical professors pursued fame rather than fortune, an ethic that mirrored contemporary developments in academe. Although an academic physician's world remained different from that of the practitioner, historian of medicine Kenneth Ludmerer has noted, their careers were, however, similar to those of academics in other fields. They sought, in the same way as their colleagues in the social sciences and liberal arts, to create high standards of teaching and scholarship and to establish their own professional spheres.[4]

The growing professional status of academic physicians during the first decades of the twentieth century incurred the wrath of practitioners, who viewed their endeavors as "impractical" and esoteric. Academics, on the other hand, perceived practicing physicians as unscientific, and their increasing professional authority eroded the established power and status of practitioners. "In their opposition to the professors," Ludmerer noted, "was all the fury, terror, animosity, and outrage of a displaced group." Academics had replaced practitioners as the heroes of the medical profession. Medical researchers by the 1920s had usurped much of the practitioners' professional authority and prestige.[5]

Clinical investigation, an academic medical specialty concerned with the application of scientific methods to the study of human disease, emerged during the decades prior to and following the

First World War. As the numbers of academic positions in this discipline increased, clinical research flourished. Those physicians, trained by pioneers in the field, had excelled at Johns Hopkins and Harvard. At these medical schools, budding clinicians learned the importance of the laboratory in making a sound and precise diagnosis. Between 1910 and 1930, motivated physicians stood a good chance of securing a full-time teaching and research position. Academic medicine, Kenneth Ludmerer has noted, had achieved complete "enthronement" by 1930.[6]

The partnership of leading American medical schools and nearby hospital facilities during the first decades of the twentieth century helped to provide appropriate clinical teaching facilities. By the First World War, Columbia University's College of Physicians and Surgeons had become affiliated with Presbyterian Hospital, Peter Bent Brigham Hospital had allied itself with Harvard Medical School, and Barnes Hospital and the St. Louis Children's Hospital had become the teaching facilities of Washington University Medical School. These institutions utilized well-trained academic physicians who understood the central place of the teaching hospital in modern medical education. So eager were the trustees of the Peter Bent Brigham Hospital and Presbyterian Hospital, for example, to insure the quality of their institution, they appointed John Shaw Billings, a central figure in the creation of the Johns Hopkins Hospital, to serve as their "expert medical advisor." The institutions that did not follow the examples of these pioneering schools soon conformed—or closed their doors—under the weight of the 1910 Flexner Report.[7]

The modern teaching hospital united the basic sciences and clinical medicine. During the 1910s and 1920s, teaching hospital-medical school alliances formed the first modern academic medical centers that offered clinicians opportunities to pursue their own avenues of research and teaching. These facilities also provided medical students and residents outstanding opportunities to hone their clinical skills. Instead of being "a way station to a pauper's funeral," as George Rosen has observed, the modern teaching hospital had become a symbol of twentieth century medicine.[8]

The Johns Hopkins Hospital became a leader in training clinical investigators. The outstanding faculty of the Johns Hopkins Medical School sought the finest medical researchers to staff its teaching facilities. This institution had already introduced the appointment of full-time faculty to its clinical departments. A generation of investigators emerged from Johns Hopkins skilled in both clinical medicine and the application of the basic sciences to their study of disease.[9]

The Boston area also provided singular opportunities for clinical investigators. By the First World War, the Massachusetts General Hospital had acquired an adequate clinical laboratory for training academic physicians. Several years later, "Ward 4" of Massachusetts General Hospital boasted patient rooms with adjacent chemical, physiological, and bacteriological laboratories. The Peter Bent Brigham Hospital also housed fine facilities to complement its staff of prominent physicians.[10]

At Boston City Hospital, the Thorndike Laboratory was also instrumental in training clinical investigators, and it produced its share of academic researchers. Of well over eight hundred physicians who were affiliated as students or professors with Harvard Medical Services and/or the Thorndike Laboratory during its first forty years, nearly half attained the rank of assistant professor or higher during the course of their professional lives. Among nearly eight hundred surviving alumni, A. McGehee Harvey noted, almost 20 percent achieved the rank of full professor, most of them in clinical medicine.[11]

In the midwest, the University of Michigan Medical School had risen to prominence. The school by the 1890s had become one of the nation's leading medical institutions. Despite its distance from the medical centers in the east and initial lack of proper facilities, the University of Michigan Medical School and its teaching hospital soon achieved a solid reputation. The Department of Medicine, for example, had attracted George Dock and other clinicians who had received their training in the finest American and European medical centers.[12]

The Peking Union Medical College (PUMC) in China also influenced the development of academic medicine. The renowned clinician Francis Peabody (who had worked at the PUMC) commented in 1922 that the unusual cases seen at the PUMC clinic provided investigators with high quality training. All patients, he added, were selected on the basis of their pedagogical and investigative purposes. To facilitate research, Peabody himself made arrangements to situate the Department of Medicine near the library, with laboratories adjacent to each ward. Regular meetings of staff and students provided a forum in which ongoing research projects and selected clinical topics could be discussed. The opportunities at Peking provided an excellent chance for aspiring clinicians to gain first-hand experience in clinical investigation. Peabody brought the same ethic of excellence to the Thorndike when he assumed its directorship in the early 1920s.[13]

Endowed research institutes also influenced the rise of academic medicine. The Rockefeller Institute for Medical Research (RIMR) and its hospital provided outstanding facilities in which investigators could conduct research on infectious diseases. The creation of this institute, combined with the strong research orientation of the nation's leading medical schools, exerted a positive influence on the evolution of clinical investigation in the United States.[14]

Whether at Johns Hopkins, the Thorndike, or other institution, each of the members of the COC felt the influence of America's finest medical centers and research facilities. During and after medical school, Committee members received clinical training at the nation's leading teaching hospitals and research institutes. By 1940, each of the individuals on the COC had also assumed prominent academic positions.[15]

Johns Hopkins Medical School influenced the careers of several COC members. Chester Keefer and W. Barry Wood had both studied there under W. T. Longcope, a leader in the field of infectious diseases. This respected clinician, A. McGehee Harvey noted, inspired numerous young students who subsequently distinguished themselves in medical research. Keefer worked under Longcope in the 1920s, and Wood was his student in the early 1930s. Longcope's insistence upon laboratory confirmation of clinical diagnoses instilled a similar ethic in both Keefer and Wood. Keefer remained at the Johns Hopkins Hospital after his graduation, serving as resident house officer from 1922 to 1923 and as assistant resident physician from 1923 to 1926. During that period he also held an assistantship (from 1923 to 1925) and an instructorship (from 1925 to 1926) in medicine at the Johns Hopkins Medical School.[16]

Barry Wood, appointed to the COC in September 1942, graduated from Johns Hopkins Medical School and later spent a summer in a clerkship at Boston City Hospital (BCH). Working in Boston under Keefer and other leaders in clinical investigation during the 1930s, Wood felt the influence of some of the nation's leading researchers. Owing to his Boston experience, Wood recalled, he was "bitten by the clinical bug." Following his graduation from Johns Hopkins in 1936, he served his internship and residency at the Johns Hopkins Hospital before accepting a research fellowship in bacteriology at Harvard Medical School. There he worked under the tutelage of the noted bacteriologist Hans Zinsser. By 1942—only six years out of medical school—he had accepted the chairmanship of the Department of Medicine at Washington University in St. Louis and physician-in-chief at its teaching facility, Barnes Hospital. Prior to his appointment to the COC, Wood had published over a half dozen papers dealing with pneumococcal pneumonia and its treatment with sulfapyridine. In these publications he had skillfully combined his interests and abilities in both clinical medicine and bacteriology.[17]

Eli K. Marshall, Jr., received both his doctoral and medical degrees from Johns Hopkins. He was awarded his Ph.D. in chemistry in 1911, and he accepted a position as an associate in physiological chemistry before receiving his M.D. in 1917. Except for a brief interlude as professor of pharmacology at Washington University in St. Louis from 1919 to 1921, Marshall remained at Johns Hopkins throughout his career. Marshall's interest in pharmacology and chemistry led him to produce important work on the toxicity of the sulfonamides in the late 1930s, the same time that Long and Bliss were also investigating the sulfonamides. Marshall's studies helped to establish clinical dosages for these drugs, and he developed sulfapyridine and sulfaguanidine, useful in treating dysentery during the Second World War.[18]

Harvard launched the careers of several other COC members. John Lockwood, for example, received his medical degree from Harvard Medical School in 1931. His record earned him a position as senior surgical fellow at the Presbyterian Hospital of Columbia University from 1932 to 1937. He had become associate professor of surgery at the University of Pennsylvania School of Medicine by 1940, the year of his appointment to the COC and its Subcommittee on Surgical Infections.[19]

Champ Lyons, one of Lockwood's classmates, forged his own illustrious career. Following an appointment as a James Jackson Cabot Fellow, Lyons graduated from Harvard Medical School in 1931. Lyons gained a wide reputation during the 1930s and early 1940s in the study of surgical infections at Massachusetts General Hospital. He used his expertise in this field to produce important work in the treatment of postoperative sepsis and was appointed to the Subcommittee on Surgical Infections in 1940. It was Lyons who conducted the pioneering penicillin work at Bushnell Hospital in Utah.[20]

The oldest member of the Committee, Francis G. Blake, graduated from Harvard Medical School in 1913 and remained in Boston until 1916 as an intern and resident at the newly constructed Peter Bent Brigham Hospital. On advice from Francis Peabody, Blake first took a year as a fellow at the Hospital of the Rockefeller Institute before working for two years as assistant professor of medicine at the University of Minnesota. Blake acquired even greater professional stature when he moved to Yale in 1921 as professor of medicine, a post he held for thirty years, and physician-in-chief of the New Haven Hospital.[21]

Blake transformed the Yale Medical School into a first-rate institution. Throughout his career, he developed an outstanding reputation as a clinical researcher in infectious diseases and, in 1931, was elected president of the prestigious American Society for

Clinical Investigation. During his thirty years at Yale, he produced important work on scarlet fever, measles, and pneumonia.[22]

The first chairman of the COC, Perrin Long, had gained valuable early experience in Boston. After graduation from medical school at the University of Michigan in 1924, Long moved east to the Thorndike Memorial Laboratory to study under Francis Peabody and work at the Boston City Hospital. The BCH gave Long solid experience in clinical investigation, and in 1929 he assumed the directorship of the Biological Division of the Osler Clinic at Johns Hopkins.[23]

The Peking Union Medical College, Rockefeller Institute for Medical Research, and the Hospital of the Rockefeller Institute also provided outstanding training for several of the COC members. Chester Keefer gained invaluable clinical experience while at the PUMC from 1928 to 1930. Calling Keefer the PUMC's "prime catch," John Z. Bowers noted in his history of the institution that Keefer worked there during its "golden decade" of the 1920s. Keefer himself remarked that his stay at the PUMC represented "two of the most productive years" of his life. Bowers also stressed that the years from 1928 to 1930 were indicative of Keefer's professional life throughout the next several decades: "A review of the publications that emanated from Keefer's two short years at PUMC shows that they characterized the high productivity that marked every phase of his outstanding career." While at the Peking Union Medical College, he published sixteen papers on a variety of clinical topics.[24]

Both Francis Blake and Perrin Long studied at the Rockefeller Institute. Blake worked at the Hospital of the Rockefeller Institute from 1919 to 1921 and was appointed to its Board of Scientific Directors in 1924, a post he held for twelve years. During his affiliation with the Institute, Blake's colleagues were among the leaders in the field of infectious diseases. "It was a period of flood tide in the clinical investigation of infectious disease," one observer noted, "and he was not alone at this stage of his life in taking advantage of it." Perrin Long also profited from his experience at the Rockefeller Institute. After studying under Francis Peabody in Boston, he joined the RIMR in 1927. Working under the tutelage of Simon Flexner and Peter Olitski, Long concentrated on the etiology of infectious diseases, an area which he pursued throughout the 1930s.[25]

Each of the COC members, with the exception of E. K. Marshall, Jr., belonged to the prestigious American Society for Clinical Investigation (ASCI). Society meetings provided an important forum for clinical investigators such as Keefer, Long, Wood, Lockwood, and Blake. The official organ of the ASCI, *The Journal of Clinical Investigation*, published some of their most important work. The American Society for Clinical Investigation allowed researchers to address improvements in medical practice "without the distractions resulting from consideration of economic, social, and political questions."[26]

Throughout the 1920s, the American Society for Clinical Investigation and its *Journal of Clinical Investigation* provided a forum in which clinicians exchanged ideas and information on their latest research projects. The Society proved especially important in the cultivation of comraderie and rapport among its members. One of its presidents noted that the Society created networks among investigators, but it also insured that only the most outstanding papers were chosen for presentation at Society meetings. Attendance at these conferences, combined with regular reading of the *Journal of Clinical Investigation*, helped to insure that interested clinicians remained at the forefront of their field.[27]

The Interurban Clinical Club (ICC), which boasted well-known clinicians from Boston, Philadelphia, and Baltimore, was similar to the ASCI in its focus. ICC members also concerned themselves with clinical investigation, and a number of them became pioneers in the field. Chester Keefer, Francis Blake, and Barry Wood, A. McGehee Harvey noted in his history of the Interurban Club, were all active members of the organization. Blake, for example, served as its secretary in 1925 and president in 1939. The Club elected Keefer, ten years Blake's junior, as its president in the early 1950s.[28]

Active in leading professional organizations for clinical investigation, the members of the COC were able to maintain close professional contacts with fellow clinicians. At meetings or through correspondence they learned of the latest research, successes, and failures of the leading physicians in the country. It was at the ASCI meeting of May 1941, for example, that an accredited investigator of the COC, M. H. Dawson, announced his early penicillin research.[29]

Common educational and professional backgrounds also enhanced the set of shared social values among the COC members. The members of the COC not only hailed from the nation's most renowned medical schools but they, just as the majority of their colleagues, were typically young and came from white, middle- and upper-class Protestant families. Physicians and medical students alike shared a devotion to the profession, respect for traditional values and religious beliefs, and common racial and socioeconomic backgrounds. These traits, David E. Rogers has concluded, made them an extremely homogeneous social group. During the years that the Harvard-trained members of the COC were working in Boston, for example, Harvard Medical School contained only a token percentage of Jews. One physician who had attended a leading midwestern medical school recalled that in his class of 120 students there were only four Jews, admitted "by quota." Available biographical data also suggest that the COC members also shared similar socioeconomic backgrounds. Perrin Long's father, for example, had been a physician, Francis Blake's father had worked as a mining engineer, and the fathers of W. Barry Wood and E. K. Marshall both had enjoyed business careers.[30]

The members of the COC were typical of twentieth century professionals with their common social, racial, and religious backgrounds. Physicians, no less than other professionals such as engineers, dentists, or lawyers, tended to be (and still tend to be) male, white, Protestant, and from middle- or upper-class families. However, COC members remained distinct from most medical school graduates during the first decades of the twentieth century. Although the number of full-time specialists had begun to increase during the 1920s and 1930s, medical students still tended to opt for general practice rather than specialization or even research as their career choices.[31]

The common social and educational backgrounds of the COC members may have influenced their participation in the wartime penicillin program and, more crucially, their relations with one another. As Harry Marks has recently suggested, the clinicians who served on the COC achieved professional stature during an important period in the history of clinical investigation. Committee members and their like-minded contemporaries championed attempts to develop "social norms and organizational controls which would ensure that a plan of study, once agreed on, would be carried out according to that agreement." Sharing similar backgrounds as well as a common perspective upon clinical research, Keefer and his colleagues could then focus their attention upon the matter at hand: the clinical investigation of penicillin according to a predetermined research protocol.[32]

Also, the members of the Committee on Chemotherapy had each studied under professors who seemed to demonstrate a single-minded devotion to medicine and were revered as the medical "heroes" of their day. The diagnostic skills and "the work habits or the utterings of these men (and they were *all* men)," Rogers noted, "were daily recounted by those who had served under them to those whom they, in turn, were teaching." Signed photographs of mentors on office walls often prompted tales of the mentors' selfless devotion to medicine. Thus, the medical greats of the early twentieth century, he concluded, profoundly influenced fledgling physicians and medical students alike. The primary "rewards" came in "prestige, respect from one's peers, and an expanding reputation as a superior diagnostician or therapist." Contemporaries of the COC members often recalled the awe and devotion inspired by their medical school professors.[33]

The accredited investigators of the COC were also well trained, and each enjoyed glowing reputations in the field of infectious diseases. Nearly half of the Committee's thirty-one accredited investigators had studied at either Columbia, Harvard, or Johns Hopkins.

All, several of Keefer's colleagues recalled, were among the most prominent infectious disease experts of their era, and they held positions at the nation's most prestigious medical schools. They represented an elite cadre within the medical profession.[34]

Although the government had called upon experts during the First World War, the use of academics such as the COC members and their accredited investigators meshed especially well with bureaucratic administration during the Roosevelt era. Early in the New Deal, Roosevelt turned to R. G. Tugwell, Raymond Moley, and other noted members of the academic community to address the nation's social and economic ills. As the war escalated in 1940, the government again called upon university-based scientists, physicians, and engineers to staff the wartime research agencies. The primary responsibility of these offices, James Phinney Baxter wrote in 1946, was "to utilize to the full the resources of the academic world." Just as physicists such as Robert Oppenheimer were logical choices for the Manhattan Project, the members of the COC were ideal as advisors on the treatment of wartime infections.[35]

Franklin Roosevelt, Barry Karl wrote, believed that the American university system could assist directly in social planning and government management. The lay public, however, displayed some suspicion of "managerial elites" who represented a trend that seemed to smack of totalitarianism. Nonetheless, academic experts had become an integral part of "the maintenance of a complex democratic system in a technological age." The decision to organize the COC and the Committee on Medical Research (the COC's contracting agency), for example, was a natural bureaucratic response to the threat of war. The individuals appointed to the Committee could then apply their knowledge and skills to the best interests of the nation.[36]

Public suspicion of elite government bureaucrats did not tend to extend to the medical profession, since magazines and newspapers had kept laymen abreast of medical advances. Novels and feature films had also showcased the tireless efforts of fictional and historical researchers alike. The popular media presented an image of beneficent, selfless physicians in the service of mankind. John C. Burnham noted, "Medicine was the model profession, and public opinion polls from the 1930's to the 1950's consistently confirmed that physicians were among the most highly admired individuals, comparable to or better than Supreme Court justices."[37]

Richard Shryock wrote that as early as the 1920s medical research had also achieved an unprecedented popularity. The *New York Times*, for example, had appointed an editor to cover medical and scientific news, and popular magazines had initiated regular features on scientific and medical discoveries. The American Medical Association even began publication of *Hygeia*, a medical monthly written for lay audiences. Periodicals, Shryock commented, provided far more comprehensive discussion of medical and scientific advances than news dailies.[38]

Novels had a similar effect on the public. Sinclair Lewis's *Arrowsmith*, published in the mid-1920s, followed the career of a young physician who, dissatisfied with life as "a regular doctor," sought cures for mankind's most deadly diseases. Denying himself, his friends, and loved ones in the interest of advancing medical science, "the drama of science obsessed" Martin Arrowsmith. The young researcher, Sinclair Lewis wrote, hoped one day "to remove pneumonia from the human race."[39]

Other works highlighted the beneficent efforts of medical researchers. Paul De Kruif's *Microbe Hunters*, published in 1926, described the heroic efforts of history's greatest medical men. De Kruif labelled one medical scientist "The Death Fighter," and he characterized another as having served both "Science and Humanity." Medical researchers, De Kruif told his readers, were a breed apart from the rest of the medical profession and lay population. Laypersons, he added, could learn of their discoveries "on the front pages of the newspapers, often before they are fully achieved."[40]

Popular motion pictures also emphasized the selfless character of the dedicated medical researcher. In the film version of *Arrowsmith* (1931), for example, the gallant researcher risked both life and love in his quest for new medical discoveries. Throughout the 1930s other feature films such as *Men in White, The Story of Louis*

Pasteur, and *The Magic Bullet* solidified the image of selfless medical men serving humanity. The cinematic portrayal of Pasteur, for example, highlighted his battle against anthrax and his role in formulating the germ theory of disease.[41]

Despite the positive public image of the medical profession, some Americans questioned the role of physicians—no matter how expert—in the rationing of a lifesaving drug. The popular notion of the physician-as-healer or the image of the kindly general practitioner stood in sharp contrast to the bureaucratic role of Chester Keefer and the COC. As one full-page story on Keefer suggested in the fall of 1943, he acted as a "judge" who cooly decided whether a patient might live or die.[42]

Many civilians, despite their objections, may have preferred to leave penicillin rationing to the impartial guidelines of the Committee. Whether consciously or unconsciously, Americans understood that the wartime bureaucracy that might *prevent* them from receiving a scarce commodity such as penicillin might also *guarantee* their access to it. In late 1942, for example, one public opinion survey found that almost 90 percent of Americans believed that the "Government should ration" scarce materials instead of citizens trying to obtain the items themselves. Another poll, taken at the height of the "rush on penicillin" in late August 1943, revealed that only 8 percent of Americans felt that "the Government" required too many sacrifices of civilians.[43]

Thus, the professional authority of the COC and its clinical investigators—bolstered by their outstanding credentials—made them the best choice for distributing penicillin to civilian patients. Had distributional decisions not been made through a system of "implicit rationing," in which a patient's access to medical services was based upon need, distribution of the drug might have been hopelessly inequitable. Patients, for example, might have received penicillin through political favor, bribery, or other means. The members of the Committee applied their expertise and training to insure the most fair and efficient method of treating civilian patients while also investigating the military applications of the drug. Until the War Production Board transferred penicillin rationing to the Office of Civilian Penicillin Distribution in May 1944, Keefer, his Committee, and its accredited investigators, all products of the nation's foremost research centers, remained the final arbiters of civilian access to "the wonder drug of 1943."[44]

Notes

1. Kenneth M. Ludmerer, *Learning to Heal: The Development of American Medical Education* (New York, 1985), 152-165, 207-233; A. McGehee Harvey, *Science at the Bedside: Clinical Research in American Medicine, 1905-1945* (Baltimore, 1978); Paul Starr, *The Social Transformation of American Medicine* (New York, 1982).

2. The most concise biographical source for the members of the Committee on Chemotherapeutic and Other Agents is Jacques Cattell, ed., *American Men of Science: A Biographical Directory* (Lancaster, Penn., 1949). For a discussion of the role of the expert in the rationing of scarce medical resources, see especially David Mechanic, "The Growth of Medical Technology and Bureaucracy: Implications for Medical Care," *Milbank Memorial Fund Quarterly* (Winter 1977): 61-78.

3. Ludmerer, *Learning to Heal*, 123-127; see also Alan M. Chesney, *The Johns Hopkins Hospital and The Johns Hopkins University School of Medicine: A Chronicle*, vols. I-III (Baltimore, 1943-1963).

4. Ludmerer, *Learning to Heal*, 130. For an excellent examination of higher education in America, see Lawrence R. Veysey, *The Emergence of the American University* (Chicago, 1965).

5. Ludmerer, *Learning to Heal*, 131.

6. Harvey, *Science at the Bedside*, xvi; Ludmerer, *Learning to Heal*, 207-217.

7. Ludmerer, *Learning to Heal*, 217.

8. Quoted in *Ibid.*, 220-224, 231; George Rosen, *The Structure of American Medical Practice: 1875-1941*, ed. by Charles E. Rosenberg (Philadelphia, 1983), 44; see also Harry F. Dowling, *City Hospitals: The Undercare of the Underprivileged* (Cambridge, Mass., 1982).

9. Harvey, *Science at the Bedside*, 183.

10. *Ibid.*, 249-273; see also Morris J. Vogel, *The Invention of the Modern Hospital: Boston, 1870-1930* (Chicago, 1980).

11. Harvey, *Science at the Bedside*, 272-273.

12. Ludmerer, *Learning to Heal*, 56-57; see also Albion Walter Hewlett, "Eight Years in the Department of Internal Medicine," *Transactions of the Clinical Society of the University of Michigan* 7 (1916): 146-149; Richard M. Doolen, "The Founding of the University of Michigan Hospital: An Innovation in Medical Education," *Journal of Medical Education* 39 (1964): 50-57; Harvey, *Science at the Bedside*, 329-336.

13. Francis W. Peabody, "The Department of Medicine at the Peking Union Medical College," *Science* 56 (22 September 1922): 318-320; John Z. Bowers, *Western Medicine in a Chinese Palace: Peking Union Medical College, 1917-1951* (Philadelphia, 1972), 122. Mary E. Ferguson, *China Medical Board and Peking Union Medical College: A Chronicle of Fruitful Collaboration, 1914-1951* (New York, 1970) also includes some useful information on the PUMC.

14. Harvey, *Science at the Bedside*, 127. The best general work on the Rockefeller Institute remains George W. Corner, *A History of the Rockefeller Institute, 1901-1953, Origins and Growth* (New York, 1964). See also Howard S. Berliner, *A System of Scientific Medicine: Philanthropic Foundations in the Flexner Era* (New York, 1985) and E. Richard Brown, *Rockefeller Medicine Men: Medicine and Capitalism in America* (Berkeley, 1979).

15. Jacques Cattell, ed., *American Men of Science: A Biographical Directory* (Lancaster, Penn., 1949) contains the most concise information on the institutional affiliations of the members of the Committee on Chemotherapeutic and Other Agents.

16. Harvey, *Science at the Bedside*, 175; Robert W. Wilkins, "Chester Scott Keefer, 1897-1972," *Transactions of the Association of American Physicians* 85 (1972): 24-26.

17. James G. Hirsch, "William Barry Wood, Jr., May 4, 1910-March 9, 1971," *Biographical Memoirs of the National Academy of Sciences* (1979): 391-392.

18. "Marshall, E[li] Kennerly, Jr.," in Martin Kaufman, Stuart Galishoff, and Todd L. Savitt eds., *Dictionary of American Medical Biography*, vol. II, (Westport, Conn., 1984), 497; Thomas H. Maren, "Eli Kennerly Marshall, Jr., 1889-1966," *Bulletin of the Johns Hopkins Hospital* 119 (October 1966): 246-254.

19. "Lockwood, John S(alem)," in Cattell, ed., *American Men of Science*, 1515.

20. "Lyons, Dr. Champ," in *Ibid.*, 1552; Henry K. Beecher and Mark D. Altschule, *Medicine at Harvard: The First Three Hundred Years* (Hanover, N.H., 1977), 327.

21. John Rodman Paul, "Francis Gilman Blake, 1887-1952," *Biographical Memoirs of the National Academy of Sciences* (1954): 3-4; John R. Paul, "Francis Gilman Blake, 1888 [sic]-1952," *Transactions of the Association of American Physicians* 65 (1952): 9-13; Harvey, *Science at the Bedside*, 293.

22. *Ibid.*

23. W. S. Tillett, "Perrin Hamilton Long, 1889-1966," *Transactions of the Association of American Physicians* 79 (1966): 59; Harvey, *Science at the Bedside*, 181.

24. Bowers, *Western Medicine in a Chinese Palace*, 77, 125; quoted in *Ibid.*, 125.

25. Paul, "Francis Gilman Blake, 1887-1952," 10; Tillett, "Perrin Hamilton Long, 1889-1966," 59.

26. Harvey, *Science at the Bedside*, 113-122; Ludmerer, *Learning to Heal*, 132-133. See also, J. Harold Austin, "A Brief Sketch of the History of the American Society for Clinical Investigation," *Journal of Clinical Investigation* 28 (1949): 401-408; Ellen R. Brainard, "History of the American Society for Clinical Investigation, 1909-1959," *Journal of Clinical Investigation* 38 (1959): 1784-1818.

27. Brainard, "History of the American Society for Clinical Investigation," 1815-1816.

28. Harvey, *Science at the Bedside*, 109-112, 122-129; A. McGehee Harvey, *The Interurban Clinical Club, (1905-1976): A Record of Achievement in Clinical Science* (Philadelphia, 1978).

29. Gladys L. Hobby, *Penicillin: Meeting the Challenge* (New Haven, 1985), 73.

30. David E. Rogers, "The Early Years: The Medical World in Which Walsh McDermott Trained," *Daedalus* 115 (Spring 1986): 2-6; Harry Marks, "Notes from the Underground: The Social Organization of Therapeutic Research," in Russell C. Maulitz and Diana C. Long, eds., *Grand Rounds: One Hundred Years of Internal Medicine* (Philadelphia, 1988), 297-336; Brendan Phibbs, *The Other Side of Time: A Combat Surgeon in World War II* (Boston, 1987), 39. Medical sociologists have also studied the socializing effect of medical education. See especially the classic monograph, Howard S. Becker, Blanche

Geer, Everett C. Hughes, and Anselm L. Strauss, *Boys in White: Student Culture in Medical School* (Chicago, 1961), esp. 435-443.

31. The literature on the history and sociology of the professions is enormous. For examinations of physicians and scientists, see especially Clark A. Elliot, "Models of the American Scientist: A Look at Collective Biography," Isis 73 (1982): 79-89; Rosemary Stevens, *American Medicine and the Public Interest* (New Haven, 1972), esp. 175-243; Magali Sarfatti Larson, *The Rise of Professionalism: A Sociological Analysis* (Berkeley, 1977), 9-63; Eliot Freidson, *Profession of Medicine* (New York, 1970); Eliot Freidson, *Professional Powers: A Study of the Institutionalization of Formal Knowledge* (Chicago, 1986).

32. Marks, "Notes from the Underground," in Maulitz and Long, eds., *Grand Rounds*, 298.

33. Rogers, "The Early Years: The Medical World in Which Walsh McDermott Trained," 2-6. On the concept of the physician as "hero," see also Philip M. Teigen, "William Osler as Medical Hero," *Bulletin of the History of Medicine* 60 (Winter 1986): 573-576.

34. "Accredited Clinical Investigators who are Receiving Penicillin: Committee on Medical Research," 23 September 1943, Committee on Medical Research Files, Record Group 227, National Archives, Washington, D.C.; personal interview with Donald G. Anderson, 5 January 1985, Magnolia Springs, Ala.; personal interview with Harry F. Dowling, 2 May 1986, Cockeysville, Md.; personal interview with Thomas R. Forbes, 13 August 1986, New Haven, Conn.

35. Barry D. Karl, "Philanthropy, Policy Planning, and the Bureaucratization of American Culture," *Daedalus* (Summer 1975): 129-149; Barry D. Karl, *The Uneasy State: The United States from 1915 to 1945* (Chicago, 1983), 113-114. See also Elliot A. Rosen, *Hoover, Roosevelt, and the Brains Trust: From Depression to New Deal* (New York, 1977); Robert Kargon and Elizabeth Hodes, "Karl Compton, Isaiah Bowman, and the Politics of Science in the Great Depression," Isis 76 (September 1985): 301-318; R. G. Tugwell, *The Brains Trust* (New York, 1968); James Phinney Baxter, 3rd, *Scientists Against Time* (Boston, 1946), 19.

36. Karl, "Philanthropy, Policy Planning, and the Bureaucratization of American Culture," 129-130, 138.

37. John C. Burnham, "American Medicine's Golden Age: What Happened to It?" *Science* 215 (19 March 1982): 1474.

38. Richard H. Shryock, *American Medical Research: Past and Present* (New York, 1947), 241-243; see also Ronald C. Tobey, *The American Ideology of National Science: 1919-1930* (Pittsburgh, 1971), 62-71.

39. Sinclair Lewis, *Arrowsmith* (New York, 1925), 323, 404; Charles E. Rosenberg, *No Other Gods: On Science and American Social Thought* (Baltimore, 1976), 123-131.

40. Paul De Kruif, *Microbe Hunters* (New York, 1926), 1.

41. Shryock, *American Medical Research*, 243-249; Jack Spears, "The Doctor on the Screen," *Films in Review* 6 (1955): 436-444; Geoffrey Perrett, *Days of Sadness, Years of Triumph: The American People, 1939-1945* (New York, 1973), 428.

42. See especially Robert D. Potter, "Heartbreaking King Solomon Dilemmas of 'Judge' Keefer," 17 October 1943, clipping in Penicillin File C39(g), Kremer's Archives, Madison, Wis.; Chester S. Keefer to A.N. Richards, 7 September 1943, Committees on Military Medicine, Committee on Chemotherapeutic and Other Agents File, National Academy of Sciences, Washington, D.C.

43. George H. Gallup, *The Gallup Poll: Public Opinion, 1935-1971*, vol. 1, (New York, 1972), 364, 406; see also F. Stuart Chapin, *The Impact of the War on Community Leadership and Opinion in Red Wing*, Community Basis for Postwar Planning Series, No. 3, April 1945 (Minneapolis, 1945).

44. For an excellent discussion of the circumvention of wartime rationing policy, see especially Richard Lingeman, *Don't You Know There's a War On?* (New York, 1972). See also Richard Polenberg, *War and Society: The United States, 1941-1945* (New York, 1972), 31-32; Perrett, *Days of Sadness, Years of Triumph*, 133-134; Deborah A. Stone, "Physicians as Gatekeepers: Illness Certification as a Rationing Device," *Public Policy* 27 (Spring 1979): 227-254; David Mechanic, "The Growth of Medical Technology and Bureaucracy: Implications for Medical Care," *Milbank Memorial Fund Quarterly* 55 (Winter 1977): 61-78; Baxter, *Scientists Against Time*, 350-353.

Chapter Three

"The Greatest Good to the Greatest Number"

The expansion of bureaucratic administration during the New Deal had helped to accustom Americans to an increased role of government in their lives. Although the final years of the Roosevelt era brought a "waning" of this trend, newly created wartime agencies still underscored the threat of bureaucracy. One contemporary writer lamented, "Congress creates a new bureau, board, commission, or authority to deal with some relatively small problem, . . . and the next thing the country knows the agency is hurling executive orders and administrative decrees to the four winds like an angered amazon." "The virus of bureaucracy," he added, "is all-pervading. It infects every organ of government." By early 1943, the wartime bureaucratic machine had swollen to include an agency to control prices (the Office of Price Administration), one to administer Japanese-American detention camps (the War Relocation Authority), and one to create policies to govern industrial production efforts (the War Production Board), to name but a few.[1]

Centralized governmental authority had attracted particular suspicion as the United States faced the worsening European situation in the late 1930s. As a result, Roosevelt directed the war effort under "widespread fears of a totalitarian future." The central problem for wartime administrators, therefore, lay in demonstrating that American bureaucracy was not antidemocratic. To administer wartime research projects effectively, OSRD Director Vannevar Bush noted, "dedicated professionals" should attempt to "combine order and efficiency without coercion." But, historian William Nelson observed, bureaucratic techniques also attempted to insure that the State functioned as an equitable provider of goods and services to all deserving citizens, regardless of their social standing or political influence.[2]

The legal and constitutional climate of the early 1940s underscored this attempt to provide all citizens with equal protection under the law. Action taken by the State, Roosevelt-era jurists stressed, must not favor one group over another. Bureaucratic distribution of penicillin represented the safest rationing system possible under the law and shielded the Committee from charges of bias. Moreover, the decisions made by the COC might well have been viewed by the courts as being actions taken by the State—a necessary point in order to activate the due process clause. The Committee operated under the aegis of the federal government and received funding from its contracts with the CMR (and its parent organization, the OSRD). Rationing of penicillin outside the COC guidelines may well have exposed the Committee to legal repercussions.[3]

A 1982 study by legal scholar Debra S. Hewetson has examined the distribution of scarce medical resources in light of the Fourteenth Amendment. In a hypothetical case brought by the relatives of a deceased patient against a hospital "allocation board," the plaintiff alleged the deceased's right to due process had been violated. The majority opinion of the court ruled, however, that the due process clause of the Fourteenth Amendment did not apply because the action of the hospital was not related to the State, and its action did not infringe upon a protected interest (i.e., life, liberty, or property) of the patient. The court continued, noting that the deceased had no legal guarantee to a scarce medical resource (in this case a donor organ). Outlining the majority opinion, one judge commented, "If we were to assume the state had a duty to provide these resources, obviously the state would have the attendent duty in developing an optimum distribution method." In his opinion, the rationing board of the hospital had allocated its resources in as equitable and "optimally rational" a manner as possible.[4]

The dissenting opinion of the court, however, reflected concerns similar to those of the COC. One judge remarked that the patient did, in fact, have a direct interest in the rationing decisions of the hospital: he died without the donor organ. "Such persons," the jurist commented, "certainly should be protected in their expectations that these decisions not be invidiously or impermissibly biased." He added that the appellant was "challenging the ultimate power of the state" to set criteria and render judgments "that one life is more worth saving than another." In this regard, legal scholar Edward Castorina has added that any rationing decisions which utilize social worth criteria "may be sufficiently questionable on equal protection grounds to overcome judicial deference to at least some legislative choices."[5]

The COC insulated itself from legal problems by adhering as closely as possible to its rationing policy. Courts since the late 1930s, legal scholar James F. Blumstein has noted, have tended to support any actions (based upon formal guidelines and carried out in a rational manner) that serve "a legitimate public interest." The Committee easily justified its actions as being in the best interest of the nation, for its research directly supported the war effort.[6]

The COC, therefore, represented but one facet of wartime bureaucratic organization—one which attempted to pursue penicillin clinical research with its policy unchallenged. The Committee exercised centralized authority, while attempting to demonstrate that its policies were equitable and in the interest of the war effort. From January 1942 until May 1944, the Committee held almost complete authority over the use of penicillin for the treatment of civilian patients. Until the War Production Board transferred rationing of the drug to the Office of Civilian Penicillin Distribution in May 1944, the unwavering guidelines of the COC yielded invaluable clinical data from an extremely limited supply of penicillin. Although the Committee produced pioneering studies of the drug's use and administration, many seriously ill civilians were refused penicillin. In the face of intense public and professional pressure to provide the drug to all who requested it, Chairman Chester Keefer stressed that a limited amount of penicillin was available only for civilians suffering from penicillin-sensitive illnesses that would yield information useful to the war effort.[7]

The COC received so few penicillin requests in late 1942 and early 1943 that Chester Keefer's task remained fairly simple. For example, the Los Angeles Breakfast Club, a prominent West Coast social organization, contacted the Committee in November 1942 to obtain the drug for one of its members suffering from osteomyelitis of the jaw. Apparently, the Eli Lilly Company had provided small amounts of the drug for the patient but withdrew it due to suspected impurities. Keefer wrote to the secretary of the club that penicillin had been used only in "the study of a few infections which are of importance to the armed forces." The scarcity of the drug did not permit extensive clinical investigation or widespread distribution. Surely the Breakfast Club understood the position of the Committee, Keefer said, adding that he regretted the shortage of the drug prevented its release in this case. When Keefer forwarded a copy of the letter to the Division of Medical Sciences, Lewis Weed replied that he was pleased that Keefer had handled matters so "effectively." Anticipating the sentiments of Keefer a year later, Weed added, "It is too bad that we must waste some of our time and energy on such matters but I see no way to avoid it."[8]

A similar request, prompted by a *Time* article in early 1943, went to the Division of Medical Sciences of the National Research Council. Philip I. Higley, a field representative of The American Dairy Cattle Club, wanted the drug for "a very valuable bull" suffering from lump jaw, a degenerative disease of the bone. Responding to his letter of February 24, W. C. Davison, the vice chairman of the Division of Medical Sciences, replied that penicillin supplies remained limited. None of the drug, he informed Higley, was available at that time for the treatment of veterinary diseases.[9]

The growing number of requests by spring 1943 prompted George K. Anderson of the Division of Medical Sciences to ask Keefer to clarify the policy of his Committee. "Could you please tell us of your usual disposal of such requests?" he inquired. "I am in doubt as to whether you provide the material or not and whether I should communicate such requests to you over the telephone or wait for the mail." Anderson wondered if Keefer even had any penicillin in his possession: "Whether you comply would seem to affect the speed of our passing on such requests."[10]

Anderson's query prompted Keefer to accept full responsibility for handling penicillin requests. He assured Anderson that he would be happy, as COC chairman, to handle petitions for the drug. "The policy of the Committee," he explained to Anderson, "has been to refuse all such requests up to the present time, the reason being that the supply is still limited. I usually write a letter to the physician explaining the situation, and that is generally sufficient." Keefer did not realize that he would soon find himself swamped with requests for the new drug.[11]

The Bushnell Hospital trials in spring 1943 convinced the armed forces of the usefulness of penicillin against serious infections. Military requirements of the drug, however, decreased the penicillin available for civilian patients. Realizing that the availability of penicillin would be severely restricted, Keefer directed the accredited investigators of the Committee to restrict the numbers of cases that they planned to treat.[12] By the summer of 1943, the Committee had used penicillin on only several hundred patients. On July 16, 1943, however, the War Production Board invoked a "freeze order," which diverted all penicillin manufactured in the United States to the Armed Forces, Public Health Service, and the Office of Scientific Research and Development (the source of the Committee on Chemotherapy's penicillin). As news of the drug's shortage reached the popular press, penicillin requests flooded Keefer's office. By April 1944, his office had received petitions from nearly ten thousand physicians.[13]

The scarce supply of penicillin for civilians forced Keefer to clarify the COC's rationing policy. The Committee divided civilian cases, therefore, into three groups: 1) cases denied the drug, 2) urgent cases with penicillin-sensitive conditions, and 3) "cases in which penicillin might be of value." Using these three categories, the Committee attempted to simplify the processing of requests for penicillin. Patients who were refused the drug suffered from conditions (such as cancer and glaucoma) against which it had no effect, and the Committee denied these cases without exception. Although the popular press had printed stories about the diseases which penicillin had treated successfully, many Americans seemed to hope that penicillin might cure nearly every malady. Faced with a grim prognosis, many patients may have requested penicillin out of desperation. Keefer's office answered these requests with a curt form letter or telephone reply, stating that they did not qualify for treatment.[14]

"Urgent" requests from patients with penicillin-sensitive illnesses prompted the most deliberation. Keefer based decisions on the severity of the case and "the type of infection." Only patients suffering from acute penicillin-sensitive conditions caused by sulfonamide-resistant streptococci, gonococci, and staphylococci were considered for treatment, and all decisions remained contingent on the availability of penicillin. The relatively low production of the drug in the United States (about 12.5 billion units per month by January 1944) did not permit treatment of all eligible cases.[15]

Dr. Donald Anderson, a research fellow in Boston University's Department of Medicine, handled civilian requests in Keefer's absence. The chairman instructed him "to find out first of all who the physician was, what hospital he was associated with, then ask him about his patient." Anderson recalled, "I'd ask him [the doctor] enough to . . . satisfy myself that. . . penicillin could be useful." He also had to determine "that the patient wasn't so far gone that there was no chance of penicillin reaching him in time." "My policy was there," Anderson commented, "and I felt it was my responsibility [in Keefer's absence] to carry it out." He added that Keefer had issued strict instructions to speak only with the patient's attending physician.[16]

Patients suffering from conditions "in which penicillin might be of value" formed the third category. According to the Committee's "Policy on Civilian Distribution," this group included "deserving requests" for which the COC hoped to release penicillin once adequate supplies of the drug became available. The majority of these cases, Keefer added, were chronic infections such as osteomyelitis.[17]

The Legal Division of the OSRD confirmed that Keefer's policy was "legally justifiable." On September 8, 1943, E. Tefft Barker of the Legal Division dispatched a memorandum to A. N. Richards (who then forwarded a copy to Chester Keefer) concerning "certain problems" that might be connected with penicillin rationing. Barker's memo reminded Richards that all penicillin research remained subject to the conditions of government contracts. "Because the effect of this rigid control has been to cut off any supply of penicillin that might otherwise have been available for civilian use," Barker wrote, "appeals are frequently made to CMR requesting it to release a portion of its allocation for use in an urgent civilian case." Since these cases did not always fit into the clinical investigative program, questions had arisen "as to whether OSRD may use the funds, appropriated to it by Congress for 'necessary expenses', for such purposes."[18]

Barker next outlined the points of executive orders which pertained to the distribution of penicillin. The OSRD, he noted, held "broad powers of disposition over personal property purchased for the perfromance [sic] of OSRD's scientific or medical contracts." Although these powers were "not without limitation," they could be "fairly taken" when they facilitated the overall OSRD research program or the war effort.[19]

Mr. Barker offered several "hypothetical cases" to clarify matters for Richards and Keefer. One involved "an urgent request" for one million units of penicillin to treat a patient with "an extremely rare and little known form of blood poisoning." Since the data might advance knowledge concerning penicillin and possibily advance the war effort, Barker counseled, use of the drug would be authorized. A similar case, which involved a disease for which researchers had used penicillin and had collected sufficient data, did not qualify for the drug.[20]

Barker also warned against "humanitarian considerations" that might influence rationing decisions. If an interesting case appeared before clinicians—one which they considered only a marginal candidate for penicillin—should the patient receive the drug? He advised against treatment of this patient. "In such a case," Barker recommended, "humanitarian considerations would be the sole ground of justification . . . because the use of penicillin has no relation to the OSRD (CMR) medical research program or to the prosecution of the war." Treatment of this patient, he added, lay outside the parameters of the penicillin investigations.[21]

Provision of penicillin for a "high ranking official" of "Country X, a South American Republic," dying from a penicillin-sensitive infection, however, would most likely be justified. Use of the drug would be authorized, Barker argued, since it cultivated "cordial relations with her [the United States'] neighbors in the Western Hemisphere." He stressed that any nation "whose defense the President has deemed vital to the defense of the United States" would even qualify for sufficient quantities of the drug "to enable it to embark upon a program of medical research." If, on the other hand, the request came from "a private citizen of Country X," the petition should be denied. Use of penicillin in the latter case, Barked noted, would neither advance medical research nor the war effort.[22]

Concluding, Barker offered "certain guiding principles" designed to keep penicillin rationing free of legal repercussions. First, treatment of civilian cases remained "legally justified" whenever researchers could glean "data relating to national defense." The attending physician, however, must submit "a complete case history." Distribution, he continued, was "equally justifiable" when done in the interest of the war effort.[23]

If borderline cases arose, then they would have to meet the above criteria as closely as possible. Should, for example, a well-known entertainer—suffering from an infection which only penicillin could treat and also scheduled for a tour of military posts—receive the drug? It was necessary, Barker noted, to weigh "morale building factors, or how instrumental must one be in the war effort before the use of penicillin . . . can be considered 'necessary, appropriate, or convenient for the prosecution of the war.' These are cases," he concluded, "for which it would seem no hard and fast rule could be established in advance and unwaveringly adhered to." Such cases should be weighed according to their particular circumstances "upon the particular factual context presented with the aid of the considerations set forth above."[24]

These guidelines, Barker believed, appeared "sound and realistic." The bottom line, as Keefer himself realized, remained penicillin's ability to treat selected diseases effectively, and the subsequent data's relevance to the war effort. An investigator of Keefer's reputation, Barker noted, was "eminently qualified" to make rationing decisions. Under extreme circumstances, Barker allowed, the CMR chairman could overrule Keefer's decision. If Richards did so, however, he would be required to justify his actions before the executive secretary of the OSRD. Acting as a kind of arbitrator, this official would then determine the disposition of the case under the established criteria.[25]

Barker had a responsibility to keep the penicillin program free of legal entanglements. In practice, however, Keefer had the final say concerning the treatment of civilian cases with penicillin, and his decisions consistently meshed with Barker's recommendations. Even penicillin manufacturers required their personnel to follow this procedure without exception. In those cases where companies had provided the drug to patients prior to the "freeze order" of July 1943, Keefer made every effort to justify continued treatment. Some patients, however, had received "fantastic amounts" of penicillin and had shown no clinical improvement. He concluded, "If after a period of adequate treatment it is felt that enough material has been used, further requests are denied." Releasing additional penicillin, the COC reasoned, might mean unnecessary waste of the drug on patients whom the drug had failed to help. Keefer agreed with Barker; however, what the former viewed as *clinical* rigor, the latter saw as a matter of *legal* necessity.[26]

Keefer and his colleagues believed "centralized control of distribution" permitted the most efficient method to ration the scarce supply of penicillin. The Committee felt Keefer had "admirably administered" its "policy of civilian appeals," and "changes would be inadvisable until [the drug] is in more plentiful supply." Keefer himself emphasized that "the present policy" had provided the "maximum" clinical data with minimal quantities of the drug. Although E. C. Andrus did not want to "burden" Keefer with a flood of penicillin requests, he noted that there were great "advantages in having them handled in the same office." Centralized administration, Andrus believed, resulted in efficient processing of these petitions.[27]

Problems occurred despite attempts to place all rationing authority with Chester Keefer. The enormous amount of publicity given to penicillin and "panic cases" caused most of the difficulty. As media coverage of the drug increased during the summer of 1943, impassioned pleas came to Keefer (and others) from all parts of the nation. One highly publicized case, treated with penicillin released through the Office of the Surgeon General without Keefer's authorization, forced the COC chairman to *insist* that all panic cases be forwarded to his office. He stressed in the strongest possible terms that, in practice, his was the final authority to determine the suitability of a case for treatment. To suggest otherwise might threaten the efficient rationing of penicillin and undermine the entire clinical program.[28]

Several cases reached national attention in August 1943, but two-year-old Patricia Malone probably posed the greatest threat to the penicillin rationing program. The *New York Journal-American's* front-page headlines—second only to reports of Allied assaults on Axis positions in Europe and the Pacific—blared " '7 Hours to Live' —Scarcest Drug Rushed to Baby." A tense "minute-by-minute" photo-essay on the newspaper's gallant efforts to save the child's life followed. Not only had the army released the drug (apparently without Keefer's knowledge), but the *Journal-American* and other newspapers had questioned Keefer's authority to ration penicillin. The *New York Sun* reported, "Red tape was cut and a supply of the new drug, penicillin, over which the Army holds control, was rushed last night under police escort from the Squibb Laboratories at New Brunswick." Overriding Keefer's authority, Surgeon General Thomas Parran had approved the release of 400,000 units of penicillin from Squibb. Ironically, the little girl reentered the hospital several weeks later debilitated by her illness. Her physician admitted that in the child's weakened condition she had "a real fight on her hands." Parran's disregard for Keefer's authority may have resulted in the improper application of the drug, since the treatment of the Malone girl may well have denied other more deserving patients. Moreover, the news reports had suggested erroneously that the army controlled civilian access to penicillin.[29]

The highly publicized case of Marie Barker, a nineteen-year-old Chicagoan, also aggravated Keefer. In midsummer 1943 the teenager developed bacterial endocarditis. As one contemporary textbook noted, it was a condition for which "no form of treatment" had yet proven successful. Although penicillin had shown some promise in bacterial endocarditis, the Committee had decided a year earlier to treat no additional cases of the disease, as it was considered to be of little military importance.[30]

Barker's widely reported pleas in major newspapers and *Time* kept her story in the public eye for nearly a month. Keefer complained that the press had "used the familiar techniques for attracting publicity," including "getting the patient to write to Mrs. Roosevelt, urging members of the family and friends to write to our Committee, urging the girl's fiance in the army to do the same, and then when she died they even went so far as to say that she died because she was unable to get penicillin." In a letter to a member of the House of Representatives who had attempted to obtain penicillin for Barker, Keefer noted succintly, "The newspapers want something dramatic."[31]

The media kept the American public abreast of Barker's condition. One article, "Last Hope Dims Out: White House Can't Help Dying Girl With Drug," told her sorrowful story, complete with a picture with her mother standing next to her Chicago hospital bed. Another quoted Miss Barker: "I am told that only the new drug penicillin will save my life," she began. "Also that the Army controls the entire supply.... I do so want to live. Won't you please help me?.... I have so much to live for.... When he [her fiance, an army sergeant] has won his fight and I have won mine, we hope to marry. It is difficult for a ill-equipped soldier to win a battle," she implored. "Will you please help me to win mine?" Marie's pleas had no effect upon the Committee, which previously had decided not to treat endocarditis patients, and in late August 1943 she died.[32]

At the same time the media was portraying Keefer as heartless and insensitive to human suffering, it also was providing the public with examples of circumventing Committee policy. Such reporting touched off a rash of pleas for the drug. Between July and September 1943 alone, the number of requests for penicillin more than doubled (see Table 3-1). On September 7, 1943, Keefer wrote a long letter to Richards about these increasing numbers. "It is my fear," he began, "that certain things which the news people are doing may not reflect [well] on the committee and the program as a whole. At least, from what they print our part in the program may be grossly misinterpreted." Controlling the civilian supplies of penicillin, Keefer had grown especially weary of the enormous number of requests for the drug. His secretary recalled that the demand for the drug became so great that proper processing of the voluminous paperwork required a secretarial staff (which was constantly overworked) and separate telephone lines to answer the calls that came to Keefer's office.[33]

The deluge of penicillin requests tested both the efficiency of the Committee's rationing policy and the mettle of the COC's chairman. "What I should like more than anything else," Keefer remarked, "is to keep my name out of the papers." The badgering of ill civilians, the press, and other groups had strained his patience nearly to the limit. Despite his efforts to fend off writers of all kinds, Keefer complained to Richards that he had had little success. Politicians, clergymen, labor organizers, and state policemen—to name only a few—also hounded Keefer to release penicillin for a particular patient. Reporters telephoned him around the clock and waited for him outside his office door, Keefer complained. Moreover, numerous "interested persons" insisted on "calling him out of bed in the middle of the night." They also wrote letters to him and printed newspaper and magazine articles about him, even when Keefer had refused interviews about penicillin.[34]

Keefer had tried "to be diplomatic but firm with these people and handle the distribution of penicillin in accordance with the rules," but to no avail. He begged for the CMR Chairman's "advice and council [sic]" concerning "the ways in which these problems can be handled, or how to manage them differently." Keefer emphasized that "we must be prepared to meet this problem as it arises from time to time in the future."[35]

Although the tactics of the press and other groups wore upon his nerves, Keefer strove to enforce the policy of the Committee: to provide penicillin only to patients suffering from illnesses where data could be of potential benefit to the war effort. Statistical analysis of available requests indicates that the single most important criteria for a civilian to receive penicillin was the presence of a condition both sensitive to the drug and of importance to the war effort. Age, gender, or other factors had no effect on rationing decisions.[36]

To handle these situations better, Keefer issued on September 7, 1943, a "Memorandum on 'Panic' Cases Which Are Supplied with Penicillin." Most of the penicillin available to the Committee, Keefer wrote in the "Panic Memorandum," went only to the "accredited investigators." Supplies to "outside investigators" (physicians who "have under their care patients . . . from whom data may be obtained will add to the information concerning the whole problem of penicillin investigation") would also be available. By providing penicillin to doctors who were not trained clinicians, the COC hoped to collect a wider range of information than the data gathered from accredited investigators alone. Keefer emphasized, however, that he accepted penicillin requests only from physicians. His office had a "standard answer" for laypersons who attempted to get the drug: "We are sorry, we can only talk with your physician."[37]

In order to minimize confusion over rationing policy, Keefer formulated an official "procedure." When laypersons contacted the Committee about penicillin, Keefer told them that their physician must contact him and send "full details" of the case. The practitioners to whom the COC chairman released penicillin received a clinical chart to record the course of the disease and explicit directions concerning the use of the drug. Dismayed by the disregard of some practitioners for clinical investigation, Keefer complained that it was occasionally necessary to contact these physicians several times in order to get them to return the paperwork.[38]

If Keefer released penicillin, a form letter accompanied the shipment, indicating the amount of penicillin allocated and the date the manufacturer had dispatched the drug. The letter stated, "Enclosed you will find a requisition blank to cover this amount of material which I am requesting you to sign and return to my office as soon as you receive the penicillin." The dispatch asked that the doctor also provide the patient's name and diagnosis in order to insure proper data analysis. This process insured that the Committee could review all pertinent clinical findings concerning penicillin. Despite these safeguards, Harry Marks has suggested, it was often difficult to restrain physicians "unwilling to relinquish control of patient management to an investigative protocol."[39]

Subacute bacterial endocarditis (SBE) represented a controversial point for the COC, for some investigators refused to deny penicillin for patients with the disease. Reminding the Committee that, as of June 1942, the ten SBE cases treated with penicillin had proven "disappointing," Keefer repeated his concern with the unauthorized use of the drug for the disease by private practitioners and accredited investigators alike. Martin Henry Dawson, Keefer noted, had "treated several patients without first consulting the Committee and used penicillin which had been released to him for other purposes." "The news of this got around," Keefer informed the COC, "and several physicians persuaded Dr. Dawson to advise them about their patients and received penicillin from manufacturers who were cooperating with our committee, without authorization from us."[40]

Keefer had informed Dawson in June 1943 that COC policy no longer authorized the use of penicillin for endocarditis patients. He reiterated that the drug had not been available for this condition for nearly a year, and "the rule" remained unchanged. He refused to yield on this matter, wishing to follow explicitly the clinical investigative program. "In fairness to everyone concerned," Keefer told Dawson, "I do not see how we can grant permission for one investigator to continue to treat subacute bacterial endocarditis and refuse others. Pressure of all kinds is brought to our Committee to release penicillin for the treatment of this disease." Keefer, a seasoned clinician himself, stressed to Dawson that he clearly understood the grim prognosis for subacute bacterial endocarditis. During Keefer's first years at Harvard Medical School, the disease had killed one of his most promising students. "I know exactly how you feel in the matter and certainly no request to treat a patient who might be benefitted is unreasonable," Keefer explained. "On the other hand," he added, "these are the problems that we all have to face in this complicated situation at the present time."[41]

Subsequent research convinced Keefer that penicillin could effectively treat SBE, but at the time he wished to keep the Committee above reproach through the strict enforcement of its policy. He reminded Dawson, "Since we have been absolutely fair about it and refused to relax our ruling regarding it we have had no repercussions." Adherence to Committee guidelines remained paramount, Keefer stressed. "As soon as you establish exceptions of rules in the distribution of material of this sort," he wrote to Dawson, "then you get into all sorts of difficulties, and the administration of the whole program is open to suspicion and is likely to break down and fall."[42]

Keefer also chastised Dr. L. W. Gorham of Albany, New York, for secretly using penicillin on an SBE patient. COC member John Lockwood completely agreed with Keefer's reaction to the improper use of the drug. He believed that Gorham had treated endocarditis patients while "many patients with definitely susceptible infections" had been denied penicillin. Two of Lockwood's own pediatric patients "tragically died during the period when it was impossible to obtain the drug, and treatment was necessarily discontinued." He added, "The 1,200,000 units which Doctor Gorham had in his possession on July 11, the day one of these children died, would certainly have saved her life." "This point," Lockwood lamented, "is not raised in any spirit of criticism or personal resentment, but may serve to illustrate precisely the sort of injustice which it is hoped that the decision of our Committee would prevent." Above all, he "deplored" any deviation from Committee policy. "Although we appear to assume a grave responsibility in certain individual cases," Lockwood concluded, "it seems to me only by adhering to this course can we provide 'the greatest good to the greatest number.'" The clinical guidelines, he suggested, existed not to deny the drug to patients but to guarantee treatment for all who might benefit from it.[43]

Francis G. Blake insisted upon a slight modification of Committee policy. Although he was willing to reconsider at some future date the treatment of subacute bacterial endocarditis caused by *Streptococcus viridans*, for the time being he fully supported Keefer's decision. "The Committee," Blake wrote, "should not make exceptions for individual cases as this will obviously lead to a great deal of difficulty and lack of confidence in its decisions." From his perspective, deviations from Committee policy would undermine the credibility of both Keefer and the COC members.[44]

Although it is quite possible that humanitarian concerns motivated physicians who treated bacterial endocarditis, Keefer insisted that their actions undermined both the authority of the Committee and the equitable distribution of the drug. Moreover, as E. Tefft Barker would counsel in September 1943, deviation from established guidelines might invite legal repercussions. Keefer had denied penicillin to bacterial endocarditis patients—such as Marie Barker, whose sad tale lay before the public eye in late summer 1943—only to discover that others had in fact received penicillin. One cannot even begin to measure the pain and bewilderment of patients who learned that others were treated while they were denied the drug. He commented that some physicians had alleged that the COC had carried on "discriminatory practices." Chester Keefer had not authorized the drug for SBE cases, but he noted that since "penicillin was being obtained by some physicians and not others made the work of our Committee extremely difficult." Moreover, the penicillin had shown only limited effectiveness against the disease (primarily because of the insufficient dosages that clinicians used), since the mortality rate still remained over 90 percent. The penicillin used on these patients had been denied other individuals who might have benefitted from it.[45]

The controversy over subacute bacterial endocarditis continued to haunt the COC. It was clear, Keefer noted after visiting Dr. Ward J. MacNeal of New York City in late 1943, that MacNeal had little interest in the penicillin effort "except obtaining material for the treatment of subacute bacterial endocarditis." Despite Keefer's refusal to release penicillin, MacNeal had acquired the drug from an unnamed supplier.[46]

The tale of how MacNeal had gotten the unauthorized penicillin, Keefer explained, grew even more "extraordinary" with each telling. To begin, "a woman appeared in his laboratory with a jug filled with a liquid, saying that he might find some use for it, but that he was not to know anything about it or where it came from." Within several days, another producer informed MacNeal that if he came to his plant he might be able to obtain additional penicillin. MacNeal then received "a large number of ampoules filled with a yellow powder, unlabeled, with the suggestion that [he] might find this mysterious material useful." In this way, Keefer grumbled, the treatment of endocarditis patients continued.[47]

MacNeal's disregard for the COC's policy annoyed Keefer. MacNeal had blatantly circumvented the authority of the Committee, threatened the integrity of the investigative protocol, and had inferred that his laboratory and Dr. Leo Loewe's in Brooklyn "were the only two places in the United States where bacterial endocarditis could be studied intelligently." Astounded by MacNeal's arrogance and complete disregard for the authority of the Committee, Keefer concluded, "I personally believe that Dr. McNeal [sic] has a very deep seated emotional approach to this whole problem and a part of his reaction is due to unconscious conflicts, since... his own son died of bacterial endocarditis shortly after the last war, and he was very anxious to do something about this disease." Personal feelings, Keefer suggested (and as Barker of the OSRD's Legal Division had warned), had no place in clinical investigation.[48]

Still other clinicians questioned COC policy. One Mayo Clinic physician with considerable experience in penicillin research, Wallace Herrell, had received a supply of the drug from Abbott pharmaceuticals but after the mid-July War Production Board "freeze order," shipments ceased. Unable to continue treating patients with penicillin, Herrell contacted Keefer on August 11, 1943.[49] He reminded the Committee of his Mayo team's willingness "to cooperate fully . . . with the subsequent work which might be done with penicillin, with which we had already been working for nearly one year." Herrell had made this clear at the December 1941 meeting of the American Society of Bacteriologists, yet he believed that the COC had "ignored" his offer. Herrell was especially offended that the Committee had not selected him and his team as accredited investigators. When Keefer offered Herrell the opportunity to assist the Committee, the Mayo physician rejected the invitation because COC policy placed too many restrictions on the "productive investigation of penicillin." Herrell concluded, "I hope that some more equitable arrangement can be made whereby work here, work elsewhere sponsored by qualified, independent investigators, as well as the studies sponsored by your Committee can be continued."[50]

The investigative program of the COC, Herrell believed, stifled academic freedom. Attempting to circumvent Keefer, he contacted Committee on Medical Research Chairman A. N. Richards and enclosed a copy of his letter to Keefer. Richards's reply fully supported Keefer's belief that policy should be maintained at all costs. "If you or your clinic were given the right to obtain penicillin direct from Abbott or another manufacturer, the same right would have to be extended to any other investigator or clinic," Richards told Herrell. Unless a central authority monitored access to penicillin, "equitable distribution [of the drug] or orderly accumulation of knowledge could scarcely be expected to result."[51]

The CMR chairman was unwilling to override Keefer's authority, but he still hoped that Herrell would reconsider his decision. The exigencies of the war, Richards told him, did not permit a more liberal penicillin policy. Although he agreed that "under ordinary circumstances" there should be no restrictions on research, the CMR chairman wrote, it seemed "obvious" that the wartime necessity of rapid data accumulation required a central authority to coordinate "objectives, efforts and results." Richards added that he believed Keefer and the COC had been "exceedingly effective" in the administration of the penicillin program.[52]

Keefer showed far less patience with Herrell's complaint, and he dispatched his own reply to Herrell. "For your information," Keefer snapped, "it should be pointed out that it is not the policy of the committee to restrict the freedom of action on the part of any investigator." However, the Committee held the responsibility for the study of penicillin-sensitive illnesses of military interest. "If we had no program and permitted the treatment of all infections regardless of their nature," Keefer explained, "we would fail in our purpose of obtaining the information that is needed."[53]

The controversy surrounding Wallace Herrell's desire to employ penicillin outside the COC's investigative guidelines did not cease. Herrell next took his case to Abbott Laboratories (which had supplied his research needs prior to the summer of 1943) and other individuals outside the circle of the COC and CMR.[54]

Herrell informed Dr. George Hazel of the Abbott Laboratories Department of Clinical Research of his clash with Keefer. "I feel sure," he began, "that the best interests of scientific investigation in general cannot be served by the restrictions placed on the release of this material." Herrell believed that "freedom of action" represented the most crucial factor in research. Scientists must be allowed, he stressed, to determine their own research agenda. In Herrell's opinion the COC guidelines hindered clinical science. Other investigators (whom he refused to name), he asserted, "elsewhere and abroad" concurred with his position.[55]

Keefer apparently had bruised Herrell's ego. The Mayo researcher agreed that the COC should not make exceptions in his case, yet he complained that Keefer had "ignored" his offer to participate in the investigative program. Keefer and Herrell could not reach a compromise. Keefer offered Herrell accredited investigator status if he followed the prescribed protocol of the COC. Herrell, however, rejected Keefer's proposal. At the same time, he continued to accuse Keefer and the COC of refusing his requests and restricting his freedom as a researcher.[56]

Herrell's vacillation continued to confuse and anger Keefer. Was Herrell willing—or unwilling—to study penicillin according to COC protocol? Keefer had apprised him of "our regulations," he told his Committee, but Herrell refused the drug "under these conditions, and he told me further that he did not expect to engage in any correspondence with me concerning the matter, and that he did not want me to request our committee to make any exception in his case."[57]

Herrell had stated in mid-August that he wished no further correspodence with the COC, yet he and his Mayo supporters would not let the issue rest. On September 17, R. D. Mussey, chairman of the Board of Governors of the prestigious institute, sent an eight-page defense of Herrell's professional credentials to the chairman of the National Research Council, Ross G. Harrison. In this letter Mussey praised Herrell's sterling record since his arrival as a Clinic fellow in 1934.[58]

Mussey—perhaps as much as Herrell and his other allies—failed to grasp the real issue. Keefer had not questioned Herrell's ability to conduct research; he had refused the drug on the grounds that Herrell's work might undermine the overall investigative program. During the postwar years, Vannevar Bush would echo the same objections raised by Herrell, but in 1943 neither the CMR nor the COC could permit such free-wheeling research. "Since the conditions of his requests are so specific," Keefer quipped, "our committee has taken the position that the matter is closed unless Dr. Herrell wants to reconsider his previous position and reopen the question for discussion. At no time have we failed to indicate our willingness to cooperate with Dr. Herrell in the question of supplying him with penicillin for his work." Keefer concluded that the COC "would be the last to do anything which would prevent progress in this field," and he assured his critics that his Committee had fulfilled its "obligations and responsibilities."[59]

Herrell insisted that he was unwilling to accept any penicillin according to COC guidelines, yet he had concluded an August 18,

1943 letter to Keefer that his laboratory still remained "available to the Committee on Medical Research in connection with the problems having to do with penicillin." His letter baffled Keefer, who explained to Donald Balfour of the Mayo, "Since this statement and the others are somewhat in conflict, it is not clear to us just what Dr. Herrell would like us to do in order that the 'facilities' may be used." He concluded, "I am writing to suggest that if you are willing to tell our committee what modifications [in the penicillin program] would meet with your approval, every possible consideration will be given to them."[60]

The matter finally subsided with Ross Harrison's letter to R. D. Mussey. Responding to Mussey's letter of September 17, Harrison expressed the hope that any ill will between the National Research Council and the Mayo Clinic had subsided. He was unwilling to supersede Keefer's original position: the matter of research protocol and penicillin rationing remained the responsibility of the COC. He told Mussey, "The differences between Dr. Herrell and the Committee concerns the reasonableness of the restrictions placed by the Committee on the use of penicillin allotted by them for research purposes, a question which, of course, I am not competent to decide."[61]

The policy of the COC, much to the aggravation of Herrell and other clinicians, reflected a growing trend in "cooperative research." The Committee required that its clinical investigators study penicillin according to a predetermined investigative protocol in order to insure uniformity of research methods and results. Furthermore, large groups of experienced clinicians, such as the COC and its team of accredited investigators, helped to guard against the possibility of bias on the part of a single researcher. Physicians such as Herrell, Dawson, or MacNeal, Keefer believed, might undermine both Committee credibility and the investigative program as a whole. As Harry Marks has observed, this problem had occurred in wartime clinical trials on syphilis. Too many physicians deviated from the predetermined research protocol and subsequently threatened proper data collection. Marks noted, "Nearly half the cases accumulated during the war had to be discarded due to incomplete information or failure to follow the protocol."[62]

Politicians also criticized Keefer and the policy of the COC. One incident involved the fall 1943 death from " 'virus' pneumonia" of Norris Higgins, a twenty-nine-year-old physician from Norwich, Connecticut. Keefer explained that "past experience" with this type of respiratory infection had proven "so unsatisfactory" that the Committee had decided to deny penicillin for its treatment. Although Keefer asked that the attending physician keep him informed of the patient's progress, his office "heard no more about the case." Instead, the Higgins family asked Senator Francis Maloney to intercede and pressure the Committee on Medical Research. The CMR, however, told him that nothing more could be done if Keefer had "all the details." "Senator Maloney," Donald Anderson recalled, "wanted Dr. Richards to use his influence with Dr. Keefer."[63]

Higgins' family and friends were convinced that penicillin would have cured the young physician. On October 22, former Congressman William Fitzgerald somberly informed Senator Maloney that Dr. Norris Higgins had "passed away." After describing the impeccable character and high social standing of the "young doctor," he addressed the circumstances of Higgins' death. "I think it is a crime that the Health Department in Washington [sic] refused to release any of this drug for his benefit," Fitzgerald asserted, "and then I read in the paper that this drug is available for men who have been careless in their lives and have contracted a dreadful disease [such as gonorrhea] can obtain this medicine." He growled, "I know you did all in your power to help us to obtain this drug but I wish that you would inform the proper officials at Washington of the way that not only Doctor Higgins's family feels about the matter, but the writer also."[64]

When Committee on Medical Research Chairman A. N. Richards received a copy of the letter, forwarded by Maloney's office, he reiterated that the policy of the COC remained entirely in the interest of the war effort—even the venereal disease studies to which Fitzgerald had alluded. These investigations had not only provided useful data in the treatment of sulfonamide-resistant gonorrhea, Richards explained to Maloney, they had permitted the swift return of infected personnel to their duties. The clinical data were "obtained in treatment of civilian sinners and necessarily the penicillin used was taken from a supply inadequate for the treatment of more respectable diseases." "I wonder," he added curtly, "if Mr. Fitzgerald would say that we should not have made that study."[65]

Other political figures also requested penicillin for themselves or their constituents. Richards once received a 2 a.m. telephone call from a patient's physician, followed by a request from Senator Hattie Carraway two hours later. When the second call came, Richards barked that he "could do nothing further until nine o'clock that morning; further that senatorial influence was not needed." On another occasion Secretary of State Cordell Hull telephoned Donald Anderson in the middle of the night to demand the reason that the Committee had refused a particular request for the drug. The groggy Anderson explained (as politely as possible under the circumstances) that the COC would not provide penicillin for lupus erythematosus. Hull pressed him, but Anderson held his ground: penicillin was useless against that malady. He emphasized to Hull that Committee policy specified that he deny the drug for all diseases lacking "clear evidence that it was going to be beneficial so that we could use it where it *could* be beneficial."[66]

The most common attempts to get penicillin through political influence involved letters to President and Mrs. Roosevelt, who received over 20 percent of all civilian penicillin requests. The total amount of mail for President Roosevelt alone averaged between five and six thousand letters of all kinds daily—ten times the correspondence received by his predecessor, Herbert Hoover. The enormous volume of mail required hiring a mail staff of twenty-two persons, with occasionally as many as seventy.[67]

Communications from family members and close friends went unopened to the President, while mailroom personnel forwarded all official correspondence to Roosevelt or "the appropriate presidential secretary." "All the rest," one study noted, "went to the Correspondence Section, a corps of clerks who determined where to forward mail for proper disposition." The staff routed most letters to one government agency or another. Letters requesting penicillin most typically went first to the Committee on Medical Research, then to the Division of Medical Sciences, and, finally, to Chester Keefer in Boston.[68]

The Division of Medical Sciences and Committee on Medical Research, in an attempt to reduce the COC's voluminous paperwork, sometimes intercepted requests forwarded from the White House before they reached Chester Keefer. These petitions requested penicillin for the treatment of cancer or another illness on which the drug clearly had no effect. At the height of the "rush on penicillin" in mid-1943, A. N. Richards informed a Mount Vernon, New York, woman that her ailing mother would not receive penicillin; the drug would have no effect on her condition. In another letter, E. C. Andrus of the Division of Medical Sciences told a Brooklyn patient that the scarcity of penicillin did not permit his treatment. In cases that clearly did not qualify for penicillin (such as cancer or glaucoma), the efforts of Richards and Andrus helped to lighten Keefer's workload.[69]

Many people who asked the COC for penicillin rarely offered details of their personal lives, only brief descriptions of their illnesses. Laypersons who contacted the White House, however, very often presented intimate (if not sometimes deeply saddening) accounts of their plight, reflecting their faith in FDR. As a number of authors have noted, Franklin Roosevelt embodied a unique talent for conveying a deep sense of personal concern to the American people. One study observed that when President Roosevelt asked his radio listeners to "tell me your troubles," many took his invitation to heart and immediately penned a letter to him.[70]

Writing to the Roosevelts to request penicillin, civilians emphasized several themes, but most persons recounted the patient's (or his or her family's) support of the war effort. A typical letter, written November 19, 1943, stated, "I have two sons serving Uncle Sam, one is a sergeant in the Army Air Corps and my other son is in the navy and is somewhere at sea. His ship sunk a German submarine about a month ago," one proud writer announced. She then came to the point: "Mr. President, I gave Uncle Sam two sons, could you please try and get me that new drug and save my husband?" A distraught mother, writing from Brooklyn, New York, on August 1, 1943, included a snapshot of her sons, one serving in the army, the other "confined to his bed with fevers that come about everyday." Begging Roosevelt for penicillin, she implored, "You cannot imagine how we all at home, here, and also my son who is in the United States Army, are hoping and praying that you will listen to our prayers and obtain the 'penicillin' drug." Another, with a nineteen-year-old-sister who was "real sick," made a similar plea: "I have a brother serving in the U.S. Army and my husband in the U.S. Merchant Marine. They are doing their part and I hope you can do a little for us."[71]

Franklin Roosevelt represented a final hope for many laypersons. Individuals who had been refused the drug by Keefer offered touching descriptions of their conditions to the President on behalf of their family members, themselves, or their neighbors. One senses in many of these petitions the pain and bewilderment of ordinary Americans trying to cope with their own serious illness or the malady of a loved one.

Yet, these civilians seemed confident that the Roosevelts could grant their supplications. Hadn't the government, personified by the Roosevelts, answered the pleas of the common person during the dark days of the Depression? Perhaps they could also help the sick and the suffering obtain the new wonder drug? One grief-stricken mother wrote to the President, "I am writing you because I do not know who else has the authority to help me or if you can possibly tell me where my son can get the medicine penicillin [.] [H]e has been sick four years and has been through the clinic and found to have streptococcus of the bloodstream." A Minneapolis woman implored in late November 1943, "So President Roosevelt, a word of yours to the government will help me." Another, writing on behalf of a friend, added cryptically, "I feel that you follow very closely in the footsteps of Jesus Christus, helping others, trusting in God." She continued, "It is my hope that, even though I feel sure your heart is ready to call you to prayer, you'll keep this because your fellow men made it for those who forget." Sadly, these letters sometimes took a month to reach Keefer's desk. If the request had come from a layperson rather than a physician, the chairman would, killing even more precious time, dispatch a form letter to the petitioner. This message informed the person that the Committee had denied the request or that Keefer required a letter, telegram, or telephone call from his or her physician.[72]

The presidential mailroom staff forwarded most penicillin requests to Keefer; however, Eleanor Roosevelt sometimes answered letters personally. Some cases she even followed up after they had reached Keefer. On one rare occasion, the First Lady's intercession may have helped to secure the drug for a patient. After numerous pleas to Keefer, Dr. and Mrs. Wilton Hallock in early December 1943 asked Mrs. Roosevelt to help them obtain the drug for their son, Duncan, suffering from ulcerative colitis. One of his nurses, Mrs. Hallock recalled, "felt that if I would write a short letter [to the First Lady] depicting our plight with [our] desire for our son, she might be able to use her influence with the government." The plea, she hoped, would appeal also to Mrs. Roosevelt's "mother compassion." Despite petitions to Keefer, the Hallocks explained, "the request was refused because they were not releasing it for this disease." "Won't you please see what more you can do," they pleaded, "and could you possibly call this to the President's attention?"[73]

While it is unclear whether she ever discussed the Hallock case with the President, on Christmas Eve 1943 Eleanor Roosevelt asked Chester Keefer to contact the worried parents. "Doctors think penicillin will help," she asserted. Receiving no immediate reply, the Hallocks telegrammed on the following day, informing Keefer of their frustration with the refusal of the Committee. Learning this news, Mrs. Roosevelt dispatched a short note to Keefer, "Would like to know outcome of Hallock case. Will you let me know?" He wired on the thirtieth that he had released penicillin for the treatment of the Hallocks' son. The First Lady's reply arrived four days later. Her secretary wrote, "Mrs. Roosevelt is glad that the Committee decided to try a few more cases of ulcerative colitis and that Dr. Hallock's son can have the benefit of the trial." Although Duncan Hallock survived, the disappointing results from other cases suggest that the drug probably had little influence on his recovery. Of the sixteen cases of ulcerative colitis treated during the war, penicillin had "no effect" on nine, four were "improved," and three died.[74]

The evidence suggests that the intercession of Mrs. Roosevelt may have influenced Keefer's decision to release penicillin for Duncan Hallock. In his letter on December 29, the COC chairman emphasized that treatment of ulcerative colitis with penicillin was contrary to Committee policy "on the ground that it was of no benefit, and secondly, there is no evidence on bacteriological grounds to make us believe that it would be effective." "Finally," Keefer reiterated, "due to the limited supply of the drug, when we use penicillin for the treatment of patients who have a disease which will not be benefitted by it, we are depriving another patient who has a disease that will be benefitted by it." Fortunately for Keefer, the Hallock case did not receive wide press coverage.[75]

No one ever explicitly threatened Keefer for denying penicillin for a patient, but Keefer did receive a setting of plates decorated "with hunting scenes or birds or something" from Abercrombie and Fitch after he had released penicillin to a New York patient. Keefer, however, could not accept the gift. Despite the protests of the patient's physician and grateful family members, he returned the dinnerware. Keefer refused tokens of appreciation, perhaps because of a concern that they might somehow cloud his objective approach to penicillin rationing.[76]

Although penicillin production had risen from less than a half billion units in May 1943 to nearly 100 billion units a year later, the rationing policy remained virtually unchanged. On April 12, 1944, Keefer reiterated that the primary responsibility of the COC remained the study of diseases of military interest which were penicillin-sensitive. The report added, "No penicillin is ever released unless the case is investigated to discover whether it fits into our research program and then only on condition that complete reports are returned to us when the end result is known."[77]

Of great importance to the future of the Committee was the subject of its continued role in penicillin rationing. Keefer informed COC members that the War Production Board, American Medical Association, Committee on Medical Research and other agencies were modifying the distribution of penicillin "to approved hospitals throughout the United States." Quite possibly, he added, the drug would "be allocated in proportion to the number of beds in each hospital."[78]

Although the COC continued clinical investigation of penicillin until December 1945, the War Production Board transferred civilian penicillin allocation to the Office of Civilian Penicillin Distribution on May 1, 1944. Home-front supplies of the drug, a committee of industrial and government officials had concluded in winter 1944, had grown too large for efficient rationing by Chester Keefer. Removing the responsibility of distribution from the COC, policy makers reasoned, would permit the COC to devote its full attention to clinical research without the bother of reporters or pleading civilians. Penicillin, the War Production Board ordered, would no longer be distributed by the Committee but through several thousand "depot hospitals."[79]

While responsible for rationing penicillin to American civilians, Chester Keefer sought to maintain the Committee's guidelines as impartially as possible. His objectivity and administrative efficiency, one colleague suggested, lay in the fact "that he listens and records—instead of talking himself." He added, "I have sometimes thought that the 'S' in his name stands for 'Silent'— not Scott." Perhaps his reticence also explains his aggravation with badgering reporters. Such reserve, however, may have allowed him, and Anderson by his example, to determine access to penicillin with cool precision. Keefer's medical school training, as well as his extensive experience as a clinical investigator, inculcated the necessity of scientific objectivity. Moreover, a detached stance may have permitted Keefer to shield himself from the emotional stress of making such life and death decisions, to don his "mask" of authority, as John Noonan has suggested.[80]

Undoubtedly, Chester Keefer shouldered the greatest burden. Although he sometimes delegated his authority to Donald Anderson, the responsibility for releasing penicillin remained Keefer's alone. His strict adherence to Committee policy shielded him and the COC from charges of partiality and, at the same time, detached him from the poignantly human dimension of his work. Although Keefer insisted that he and the Committee held "no power over the life or death of anyone," many laypersons believed that he—not to mention "the government," as one person told Franklin Roosevelt —did make life and death decisions.[81]

Keefer's devotion to Committee policy also streamlined the rationing process by simplifying the selection of patients for treatment. Either an individual case met—or did not meet—the objective criteria of the COC's guidelines.[82] Keefer also believed that adherence to research guidelines advanced both the war effort and cooperative clinical investigation. It is significant that Anderson and Keefer's pioneering 1948 study, based on wartime experience with penicillin, bore the title, *The Therapeutic Value of Penicillin: A Study of 10,000 Cases*. These "cases," many of which Keefer never saw, were fortunate enough to qualify for treatment with "the wonder drug of 1943," penicillin.[83]

Chester Keefer's adherence to clinical protocol helped to maintain an equitable system of penicillin rationing. If Keefer had yielded to political or professional pressure, the distribution process may have been reduced to a question of which individuals could muster the most signatures on a petition or attract the most media attention. As the cases of Marie Barker and Dr. Norris Higgins illustrate, media attention had little effect on Keefer's decisionmaking. Acting on Keefer's orders, Donald Anderson even refused a petition from Secretary of State Cordell Hull. While many civilians may have perceived Keefer as a cruel judge, he and his cadre of "dedicated professionals" played a crucial role in the equitable distribution of one of the most important drugs of the twentieth century.

Notes

1. The author would like to thank the *Journal of the History of Medicine and Allied Sciences* for its kind permission to use large portions of the author's "Wartime Bureaucracy and Penicillin Allocation: The Committee on Chemotherapeutic and Other Agents, 1942-1944," *Journal of the History of Medicine and Allied Sciences* 44 (April 1989): 196-217 on which much of this chapter is based. Richard Polenberg, *War and Society in the United States: 1941-1945* (New York, 1972), 73-98; Barry D. Karl, *The Uneasy State: The United States, 1915-1945* (Chicago, 1984), 231; Barry D. Karl, "Philanthropy, Policy Planning, and the Bureaucratization of the Democratic Ideal," *Daedalus* (Summer 1975): 129-130; Lawrence Sullivan, *The Dead Hand of Bureaucracy* (Indianapolis, 1940), 15, 17. See also Henry M. Wriston, *Challenge to Freedom* (New York, 1943); Herman Finer, "Critics of 'Bureaucracy,' " *Political Science Quarterly* 60 (March 1945): 100-112.

2. Robert Cuff, "American Mobilization for War, 1917-1945: Political Culture vs. Bureaucratic Administration," in N. F. Dreiszinger, ed., *Mobilization for Total War: The Canadian, American and British Experience: 1914-1918, 1939-1945* (Waterloo, Ontario, 1981), 74, 85-86; William E. Nelson, *The Roots of American Bureaucracy, 1830-1900* (Cambridge, Mass., 1982), 1-8, 156-161.

3. Paul S. Murphy, *The Constitution in Crisis Times, 1918-1969* (New York, 1972).

4. Debra S. Hewetson, "Scarce Medical Resource Allocation—The Case of First Impression: A Hypothetical Opinion of the Twelfth Circuit United States Court of Appeals," *Journal of Legal Medicine* 3 (1982): 295-315.

5. *Ibid.*; Edward Castorina, "Scarce Life-Saving Medical Resources: Equal Protection and Patient Selection," *Journal of Legal Medicine* 1 (July 1979): 154-179.

6. James F. Blumstein, "Rationing Medical Resources: A Constitutional, Legal, and Policy Analysis," *Texas Law Review* 59 (November 1981): 1345-1399.

7. See especially James Phinney Baxter, *Scientists Against Time* (Boston, 1946), 350-351; Chester S. Keefer, "Penicillin: A Wartime Accomplishment," in E.

"The Greatest Good to the Greatest Number" 95

C. Andrus et al., eds., *Advances in Military Medicine Made by American Investigators Working Under the Sponsorship of the Committee on Medical Research*, vol. II, Science in World War II, Office of Scientific Research and Development Series (Boston, 1948), 719-722; Donald G. Anderson and Chester S. Keefer, *The Therapeutic Value of Penicillin: A Study of 10,000 Cases* (Ann Arbor, Mich., 1948), iii-vii.

8. Chester S. Keefer to the Secretary, Los Angeles Breakfast Club, 20 November 1942; Chester S. Keefer to Lewis H. Weed, 20 November 1942; Lewis H. Weed to Chester S. Keefer, 24 November 1942, Committees on Military Medicine Files, Committee on Chemotherapeutic and Other Agents, National Academy of Sciences, Washington, D.C. [Hereafter cited as COMM, NAS]. The War Production Board did not completely control penicillin production until July 16, 1943. See especially Gladys L. Hobby, *Penicillin: Meeting the Challenge* (New Haven, 1985): 171-197.

9. P. I. Higley to National Research Council, 24 February 1943; W. C. Davison to P. I. Higley, 1 March 1943, COMM, NAS.

10. George K. Anderson to Chester Keefer, 27 February 1943, COMM, NAS.

11. Chester S. Keefer to George K. Anderson, 4 March 1943, COMM, NAS.

12. Chester S. Keefer, "Memorandum on Penicillin Distribution," 25 May 1943, Committee on Medical Research Files, Record Group 227, National Archives, Washington, D.C. [Hereafter cited as CMR, RG 227.]

13. "Allocation Order M-338," 9 July 1943, CMR, RG 227.

14. Penicillin Producers, Industry Advisory Committee: Summary of Meeting, 22 September 1943, 4-5, CMR, RG 227; "Public Vies With Army for Penicillin, Miracle Drug That Comes From Mold," *Newsweek*, 30 August 1943, 68.

15. *Ibid.*

16. Personal interview with Donald G. Anderson, 5 January 1985, Magnolia Springs, Ala.

17. Penicillin Producers, Industry Advisory Committee: Summary of Meeting, 22 September 1943, 5, CMR, RG 227.

18. John T. Connor to A. N. Richards, 8 September 1943, CMR, RG 227; E. Tefft Barker to John T. Connor, 3 September 1943, CMR, RG 227.

19. Barker to Connor, 3 September 1943, CMR, RG 227.

20. *Ibid.*

21. *Ibid.*

22. *Ibid.*

23. *Ibid.*

24. *Ibid.*

25. *Ibid.*

26. Committee on Chemotherapeutic and Other Agents, Minutes of Meeting, 20 August 1943, COMM, NAS; see also Chester S. Keefer to A. N. Richards, 7 September 1943, CMR, RG 227.

27. *Ibid.*; E. C. Andrus to Chester S. Keefer, 26 June 1943, CMR, RG 227.

28. *Ibid.*

29. Charles Davis, " '7 Hours to Live'—Scarcest Drug Rushed to Baby," *New York Journal-American*, 12 August 1943, 1; "A Stirring Race to Save a Baby's Life As Hope Rode upon the Hands of a Clock," *New York Journal-American*, 12 August 1943; "Penicillin Breaks Red Tape to Save Child's Life Here," *New York Sun*, 12 August 1943; "Army Releases Rare Penicillin to Save Life of Queens Girl, 2," *New York Herald-Tribune*; "Girl Once Saved by Penicillin Is in Critical Condition," n.s., 15 September 1943. All clippings in CMR, RG 227.

30. Marie Barker probably received the greatest single amount of national media coverage of all civilians who requested penicillin from the Committee on Chemotherapy. One of the first reports of her condition appeared in "Rush on Penicillin," *Time*, 30 August 1943, 44-46. See also the following clippings, available in Penicillin File C39 (g), Kremer's Reference Files, University of Wisconsin, Madison, Wis. [hereafter cited as KRF]: "Uncle Appeals to President for Penicillin for Girl," *The Evening Star* [Washington, D.C.], 17 August 1943; "Stricken Girl Begs First Lady for Penicillin," [*Washington?*] *Times-Herald*, 17 August 1943; "Penicillin Helps Boy; Is Denied Woman," *The Evening Star*, 18 August 1943; "Chicago Girl Loses Fight Against Blood Disease," n.s., 26 August 1943. The clipping, "Last Hope Dims Out," is available in CMR, RG 227. Russell L. Cecil, ed., *A Textbook of Medicine* (Philadelphia, 1944), 1076; [Chester Keefer], "Memorandum to the Committee on Chemotherapeutic and Other Agents on Penicillin and the Treatment of Bacterial Endocarditis," December 1943, CMR, RG 227.

31. Chester S. Keefer, "Memorandum on the Case of Marie Barker," n.d.; Chester S. Keefer to Eugene Worley, 13 September 1943, CMR, RG, 227.

32. "Last Hope Dims Out," CMR, RG 227; "Stricken Girl Begs First Lady for Penicillin," KRF; "Chicago Girl Loses Fight Against Blood Disease," KRF.

33. Chester S. Keefer to A. N. Richards, 7 September 1943, CMR, RG 227; personal interview with Constance Haynes MacDonald, 29 May 1985, Boston, Mass.

34. Chester S. Keefer to A. N. Richards, 7 September 1943, CMR, RG 227; Marie O'Brien, "Penicillin Use, Supply Limited, Guardian Warns," *Washington Times-Herald*, 24 October 1943, CMR, RG 227.

35. *Ibid.*

36. The statistical test employed, r-phi, yielded a value of .51 when granting of a request was compared to the presence of the reported condition on the program of the Committee. Controlling for the patient's residence near an accredited investigator (r-phi=0), writing to Chester Keefer (r-phi=.18), before and after January 1944 (r-phi=-.28), writing to Franklin Roosevelt (r-phi= -.15), and population of community (r-phi=-0.6) yielded a much weaker statistical relationship. The high value (r-phi = .51) suggests that presence of an illness on the clinical guidelines of the Committee represented the most important criterion for the granting of a civilian request. The data (N=211) for this analysis were taken from CMR, RG 227.

37. Chester S. Keefer to A.N. Richards, 7 September 1943, "Memorandum on 'Panic' Cases Which Are Supplied Penicillin," CMR, RG 227.

38. *Ibid.*

39. Chester S. Keefer to E. C. Andrus, 14 December 1943, CMR, RG 227; Harry M. Marks, "Notes from the Underground: The Social Organization of Therapeutic Research," in Russell C. Maulitz and Diana E. Long, eds., *Grand Rounds: One Hundred Years of Internal Medicine* (Philadelphia, 1988), 299.

40. [Chester S. Keefer], "Memorandum to the Committee on Chemotherapeutic and Other Agents on Penicillin and the Treatment of Bacterial Endocarditis," December 1943, 1, CMR, RG 227.

41. Chester S. Keefer to M. H. Dawson, 12 June 1943, CMR, RG 227. The death in 1931 of Harvard medical student Alfred Reinhart is mentioned in Wesley W. Spink, *Infectious Diseases: Prevention and Treatment in the Nine-*

teenth and Twentieth Centuries (Minneapolis, 1978), 272-273. See also Soma Weiss, "Self-Observations and Psychologic Reactions of Medical Student A.S.R. to the Onset and Symptoms of Subacute Bacterial Endocarditis," *Journal of the Mount Sinai Hospital* 8 (1941-1942): 1079-1094.

42. *Ibid.*; Donald G. Anderson and Chester S. Keefer, "Treatment of Nonhemolytic Streptococcus Subacute Bacterial Endocarditis with Penicillin," *Medical Clinics of North America* 29 (September 1945): 1129.

43. Chester S. Keefer to L. W. Gorham [n.d., probably summer 1943]; John S. Lockwood to Chester S. Keefer, 12 August 1943, CMR, RG 227.

44. Francis G. Blake to Chester S. Keefer, 11 August 1943, CMR, RG 227. As increased supplies of penicillin permitted treatment of bacterial endocarditis patients (and additional clinical studies showed the effectiveness of the drug in those cases), Keefer and the Committee in 1944 allowed study of these cases. See especially, Hobby, *Penicillin: Meeting the Challenge*, 161-170; Paul De Kruif, "Conquest of a Killer," *Reader's Digest*, March 1945, 27-31; Paul De Kruif, *Life Among the Doctors* (New York, 1949), 211-245.

45. [Chester S. Keefer], "Memorandum ... on Bacterial Endocarditis," December 1943, 2-3, CMR, RG 227.

46. [Chester S. Keefer], "Memorandum to Dr. A. N. Richards Concerning Visit with Dr. Ward J. McNeal, New York City," December 1943, 1, CMR, RG 227.

47. *Ibid.*, 2.

48. *Ibid.*

49. Wallace E. Herrell to Chester S. Keefer, 11 August 1943, CMR, RG 227.

50. *Ibid.*

51. A. N. Richards to Wallace E. Herrell, 13 August 1943, COMM, NAS.

52. *Ibid.*

53. Chester S. Keefer to Wallace E. Herrell, 16 August 1943, COMM, NAS.

54. Wallace E. Herrell to George R. Hazel, 4 September 1943, CMR, RG 227.

55. *Ibid.*

56. *Ibid.*

57. *Ibid.*

58. R. D. Mussey to Ross G. Harrison, 17 September 1943, CMR, RG 227.

59. Chester S. Keefer to S. DeWitt Clough, 13 September 1943, COMM, NAS.

60. Chester S. Keefer to Donald C. Balfour, 28 September 1943; Chester S. Keefer to Ross G. Harrison, 28 September 1943, COMM, NAS.

61. Ross G. Harrison to R. D. Mussey, 2 October 1943, COMM, NAS.

62. Marks, "Notes from the Underground," in Maulitz and Long, eds., *Grand Rounds*, 310-311.

63. "Memorandum: Telephone Conversation with Dr. Anderson re: Dr. Norris Higgins," 15 November 1943; "Record of Call of October first [1943], CMR, RG 227.

64. William Fitzgerald to Francis Maloney, 22 October 1943, CMR, RG 227.

65. A. N. Richards to Francis Maloney, 17 November 1943, CMR, RG 227.

66. A. N. Richards to Chester S. Keefer, 29 November 1943, COMM, NAS; personal interview with Donald G. Anderson.

67. The percent of requests to Franklin Roosevelt is based upon a sample of allocation requests (N=211) found in the Committee on Medical Research Files, RG 227; Leila A. Sussmann, "FDR and the White House Mail," *Public Opinion Quarterly* 20 (Spring 1956): 5-6.

68. *Ibid.*, 6; Chester S. Keefer to E. C. Andrus, 14 December 1943, CMR, RG 227.

69. A. N. Richards to Gladys Watt, 24 September 1943; E. C. Andrus to Jack Hunter, 5 November 1943, CMR, RG 227.

70. For examinations of Franklin Roosevelt's public image, see especially James M. Burns, *Roosevelt: The Soldier of Freedom* (New York, 1970); Arthur Schlesinger, Jr., *The Age of Roosevelt: The Crisis of the Old Order* (New York, 1957) and *The Coming of the New Deal* (New York, 1959); William E. Leuchtenberg, *Franklin D. Roosevelt and the New Deal* (New York, 1963); Sussmann, "FDR and the White House Mail," 10. See also Fillmore H. San-

ford, "Public Orientation to Roosevelt," *Public Opinion Quarterly* 15 (Summer 1951): 189-216.

71. Mrs. Fabry [?] to Franklin Roosevelt, 19 November 1943; Philomena Ribis to Franklin Roosevelt, 1 August 1943; Mrs. Charles E. Martin to Franklin Roosevelt, n.d., CMR, RG 227.

72. Mrs. Minnie Edgecomb to Franklin Roosevelt, 7 September 1943; Mrs. Marie Carlson to Franklin Roosevelt, 24 November 1943; Miss Charlene Joy Farrand to Franklin Roosevelt, 2 December 1943, CMR, RG 227.

73. Wilton Hallock to Eleanor Roosevelt, 21 December 1943, Eleanor Roosevelt Collection, FDR Library, Hyde Park, New York. [hereafter cited as ERC]. Hortense Hallock to David P. Adams, 28 August 1986, in personal files of David P. Adams, Department of Humanities, Columbus State Community College, Columbus, Ohio; Arthur Bloomfield, "Diseases of the Alimentary Tract," in John H. Musser, ed., *Internal Medicine: Its Theory and Practice in Contributions by American Authors*, 2nd rev. ed. (Philadelphia, 1934), 642.

74. Eleanor Roosevelt to Chester S. Keefer, 24 December 1943; Eleanor Roosevelt to Chester S. Keefer, 29 December 1943; Chester S. Keefer to Eleanor Roosevelt, 30 December 1943; Secretary to Mrs. Roosevelt [Malvina Thompson?] to Chester S. Keefer, 3 January 1944, ERC; telephone interview with Duncan Hallock, 9 August 1986; Anderson and Keefer, *The Therapeutic Value of Penicillin*, 281.

75. Chester S. Keefer to Eleanor Roosevelt, 29 December 1943, ERC.

76. Personal interview with Donald G. Anderson, 5 January 1985.

77. Kenneth B. Raper, "A Decade of Antibiotics in America," *Mycologia* 44 (January-February 1952): 41; Robert D. Coghill and Roy S. Koch, "Penicillin: A Wartime Accomplishment," *Chemical and Engineering News* 23 (25 December 1945): 2310; "Committee on Chemotherapy, Minutes of Meeting," 12 April 1944, 1, COMM, NAS.

78. "Committee on Chemotherapy, Minutes of Meeting," 12 April 1944, 14, COMM, NAS.

79. Anderson and Keefer, *The Therapeutic Value of Penicillin*, iii-viii; Hobby, *Penicillin: Meeting the Challenge*, 143-144; Baxter, *Scientists Against Time*, 350.

80. A. Baird Hastings, "Chester Scott Keefer, M.D., D.Sc.: Physician and Teacher, Extraordinary," *The Boston Medical Quarterly* 14 (September

1963): 90; John T. Noonan, Jr., *Persons and Masks of the Law* (New York, 1976), 19-21. See also J. C. Duffy, *Emotional Issues in the Lives of Physicians* (Springfield, Ill., 1970).

81. Chester S. Keefer, "Memorandum on the Case of Marie Barker," n.d., CMR, RG 227.

82. Anderson and Keefer, *The Therapeutic Value of Penicillin*. The issue of "physician as gatekeeper" has been discussed in Deborah A. Stone, "Physicians as Gatekeepers: Illness Certification as a Rationing Device," *Public Policy* 27 (Spring 1979): 227-254.

83. Anderson and Keefer, *The Therapeutic Value of Penicillin*.

Chapter Four

A "Rush on Penicillin"

Media coverage of penicillin in the latter half of 1943 sparked a flood of civilian requests for the drug. While A. N. Richards believed that these sensationalized (and often inaccurate) news reports fueled an insatiable demand for penicillin, Chester Keefer felt that journalists threatened the credibility of the COC and its rationing policy. Only in the case of classified production information and when dealing with the Office of War Information (OWI) and private filmmakers did Richards and Keefer succeed in censoring popular reports about penicillin. Journalists, unwilling to follow OWI attempts to control public information or accept the tight-lipped stance of Keefer and Richards, filled major newspapers and magazines with stories of patients whom the drug had miraculously saved. At the same time, advertising executives tied penicillin directly to the war effort by couching the drug in military imagery. Only in mid-1944, when adequate supplies of the drug existed to satisfy a greater number of civilian requests, did the COC and CMR cease their attempts to limit the widespread publicity of the drug. By that time, however, the media had created a huge market for penicillin.[1]

Richards and Keefer first clashed with the media in late 1942 when the press discovered that some of Boston's Coconut Grove burn victims had received the new drug. Reporters, Keefer explained to Richards, learned of the use of penicillin "somewhere at the Massachusetts General Hospital as the result of a Surgical Staff Conference, at which [the staff] discussed the treatment of burns from the Cocoanut [sic] Grove Disaster." Keefer was quick to emphasize that he had not leaked the information.[2]

In the aftermath of the Coconut Grove fire, Keefer directed inquisitive reporters to A. N. Richards, since a CMR contract had supplied the penicillin. Richards, however, was reluctant to discuss penicillin use with the press; too little of the drug existed to risk exciting the public. When Jean Pinanski, a *Boston American* reporter, pressured him about a "human interest" story on it, Richards curtly refused her request. He stressed that neither the CMR nor the COC wished "to encourage a national demand until there is some prospect of being able to supply it [penicillin]." Richards told another journalist who wanted "first crack at penicillin" that he disapproved of widespread publicity of the drug. He added that raising "hopes in the minds of suffering individuals which cannot be satisfied would . . . be unjustifiable." After Lawrence Dame of the *Boston Herald* hounded Richards for information on penicillin, Richards reiterated, "The distress which would thus be caused seems to me far to outweigh any possible advantage which might be gained by the publication of a story at the present time." He hoped that Dame would not pursue the matter. Despite Richards's efforts, the *Herald* announced, "Penicillin came through the disaster test with flying colors, as demonstrated by the absence of infections in the burns of those treated with it."[3]

No attempt was made to discourage publicity of the sulfa drugs, however. The public, after all, had known of the sulfonamides for several years. In November 1942, for example, Eleanor Bliss, a sulfonamide expert from Johns Hopkins, received an offer from the Lord and Thomas Advertising firm to do an educational broadcast on the sulfonamides. On the condition that the broadcast included no references to the Committee on Medical Research or Office of Scientific Research and Development, E. C. Andrus told Bliss that a discussion of the sulfas' role in the war effort seemed timely. Unlike penicillin, the sulfa drugs remained in ample supply. Furthermore, reports on the sulfonamides might even have diverted public attention from penicillin.[4]

Penicillin in the summer of 1943 began to attract increasing public attention. By this time, researchers had treated several hundred patients with the drug and demonstrated its usefulness against a number of infections. The new "wonder drug of 1943" seemed to surpass even the sulfonamides. "Once the news media realized what penicillin was...," one writer observed, "it became increasingly difficult to force the genie back into the lamp." Only on rare occasions, when journalists allowed the CMR to approve their stories, was Richards able to control reports about the drug, insuring that stories be both factual and within security guidelines. When *Liberty*'s Edward Hutchings, Jr., submitted an article for Richards's consideration in June 1943, the CMR chairman bristled. Hutchings's "prediction" that penicillin might surpass the sulfas, Richards stated, "even should it come true, is completely unjustified at the present time." In light of existing studies, he told the reporter, few researchers believed that penicillin would replace the sulfonamides.[5]

Richards may well have been stalling the inquisitive reporter. Several weeks prior to his correspondence with Hutchings, Richards had authored the official CMR statement on the drug published in the *Journal of the American Medical Association*. This short piece had outlined penicillin's history, its use in serious infections, and its extreme scarcity. Moreover, Chester Keefer had kept Richards abreast of Champ Lyons's successes at Bushnell Hospital throughout April 1943. As chairman of the Committee on Medical Research, he was well aware of penicillin's potential.[6]

Hutchings's assertions that "Washington" had finally "broken down and confessed" also annoyed Richards. The CMR chairman chided, "If by Washington you mean the National Research Council and the Committee on Medical Research, you may be assured that there has been no effort to keep the virtues of penicillin hidden" from the American public. He added, however, that reports about the scarce drug's curative powers only exacerbated the "suffering and despair in the hearts of those whom it could conceivably benefit." Moreover, Richards considered allegations of a cover-up to be "unfair."[7]

It was not surprising that Richards was often unable to regulate reports on penicillin. Story-hungry wartime journalists, one study noted, grew uncomfortable with official attempts to control "what news could be printed and what should be withheld," as the Committee on Public Information had done during the First World War. Reporters increasingly ignored wartime agencies that attempted to censor the news releases. Far better, one wartime columnist retorted, "that the public should be confused temporarily than that opposing viewpoints should be muffled or suppressed."[8]

Although reporters may have felt justified in exercising the freedom of the press, their zeal complicated penicillin rationing by confusing the American public. Some stories in summer 1943 stated that only Chester Keefer could release the drug; other accounts described how seriously ill civilians somehow had received the drug from the army. In September 1943, the *New York Times* reported the case of an eleven-year-old girl at the Hadassah University Hospital in Jerusalem. The patient, suffering from a severe infection, recovered when the Army Medical Corps treated her with the drug. A similar story described the case of Anne Shirley Carter, a fifteen-year-old patient at Middle Georgia Hospital in Macon. The teenager had qualified for penicillin, "but by error it was mailed parcel post." When the army learned of the mistake, the *Times* wrote, the military flew a "1,000 mile mercy errand" to deliver the drug to the young girl. The author of the article, however, failed to mention Keefer's role in releasing the penicillin. The heavy publicity in the *New York Journal-American* about Patty Malone—for whom the surgeon general had reportedly released the drug—had also bred confusion about rationing policy.[9]

When the headline "Army to Get Its Magic Penicillin, Needs 5 Billion Units Weekly" appeared on the front page of the *New York Herald Tribune* on July 30, 1943, one of A. N. Richards's colleagues wrote sarcastically in a memo, "Newt—Good morning. Hope you are feeling fine and up to anything (read this)." An "unauthorized source" from Winthrop Chemicals, he noted, had leaked the delicate information to the press. Another colleague, underscoring a report about the army's particular interest in gonorrhea, joked to the CMR chairman, "Hold on to your hat!!"[10]

The media also emphasized (correctly this time) that the armed forces received most of the penicillin produced in the United

States. Popular articles such as "'Wonder Drug' Pencillin [sic] Brings Magic Healing to Army," "Penicillin: New Wonder Drug from Mold," and "Restoring War Victims" described the crucial role that penicillin played in the treatment of wounded soldiers. One report announced that the new drug had already saved thousands on the battlefront. One pictured an army nurse administering "a 'shot' of the precious penicillin" to a soldier wounded in the Kasserine Pass. Another article credited penicillin with saving the life of an infantryman "who tripped over a German land mine in Sicily." The *New York Times* even dubbed Ian Fraser, a British lieutenant colonel, a "pioneer" in the history of penicillin. Fraser, the *Times* reported, had received a Distinguished Service Order (DSO) commendation for administering the drug to wounded soldiers "under heavy enemy fire on the Sicilian Beaches." His DSO citation boasted that the brave officer had "used technique novel to war surgery and most valuable wound treatment [sic]."[11]

Mona Gardner's "Miracle from Mold," published in the September 1943 *Women's Home Companion*, also touted the drug as an amazing cure-all and presented vignettes of military personnel whom the drug had saved. The armed forces, Gardner explained, recognized penicillin as a "powerful weapon" in the war against battlefield infections. Although "yesterday's wonder drugs, the sulfa compounds, . . . merely slow up bacterial growth," she explained, "penicillin is a killer. At least fifteen virulent bacterial strains which have remained toughly resistant to the sulfonamides have gone down when exposed to penicillin's onslaught." The story's caption announced, "Everybody with a husband, son or sweetheart in the armed forces will thrill to the story of penicillin—a new germ-killer acclaimed as more potent than the fabulous sulfa drugs."[12]

Although these reports about penicillin fueled the civilian demand for the drug, the press had emphasized that huge military requirements of penicillin severely reduced home-front supplies. Colonel Paul Robinson of the Army Medical Corps stated that by mid-September the army alone would require nearly five billion units per week. A *New York Times* article explained to civilians that penicillin remained "under strict allocation" by the War Production

Board in the interest of national defense; there was little hope that surplus supplies would soon be available. Production levels remained "a military secret," but the report added that army and navy medical personnel hoped to "save thousands of lives among our wounded and sick fighting men."[13]

The army felt that these reports suggested that it controlled—if not stockpiled—penicillin. A. N. Richards cautioned the Department of Agriculture's C. F. Speh, who had been asked to participate in a broadcast about his agency's role in penicillin research, to avoid suggestions that the armed forces received "every grain of penicillin." The military, he added, did not wish "to be accused of depriving the civilian population entirely of all the drug." The Office of the Surgeon General noted in August 1943, "Publicity on penicillin has been most unfortunate in two particular respects." First, the popular press had suggested that the "miracle drug" was a panacea which researchers "understood thoroughly." "Second, and even more regrettable," the memorandum added, "is the misconception that the Army controls the entire supply of penicillin."[14]

The Office of the Surgeon General, also concerned about the reports, asked A. N. Richards in late July 1943 to issue a press release to the Associated Press. The surgeon general hoped that this statement would clarify the public perception of rationing and production efforts. However, the release never received extensive media coverage. When Keefer questioned why most newspapers had ignored the story, one journalist snapped that "no newspaper wants to tell people about something that is scarce and that they can't get." "In other words," Keefer replied, "there is nothing dramatic about a factual, earnest statement insofar as penicillin production and distribution is concerned."[15]

News of the penicillin scarcity touched off "a wave of frantic appeals" in the summer of 1943. *Time*, referring to recent reports on the drug, wrote on August 30 that "the wonder drug of 1943 last week made headlines up and down the nation." *Newsweek* announced on the same day, "Public Vies With Army for Penicillin, Miracle Drug That Comes From Mold." The lead of the article asked, "When there is only enough of the newest miracle drug to save either a child or wounded soldier, which one would you save?" "Last week," *Newsweek* explained, "this poser stumped the nation." Focusing upon "the drug that brought the question of soldier or civilian survival into sharpest conflict," the periodical reiterated that "all pleas for the germ destroyer would be passed along to Dr. Chester S. Keefer."[16]

In trying to clarify penicillin rationing policy, the popular press thrust Chester Keefer into the public eye. The *New York Times*, for example, stressed that he alone controlled civilian penicillin and acted "for Dr. A. N. Richards, Chairman of the Committee on Medical Research of the Office of Scientific Research and Development." Physicians who tried to obtain penicillin for their patients, newspapers announced, were required to "submit complete medical and bacteriological case histories to Dr. Chester S. Keefer chairman of the Committee on Chemo-Therapy [*sic*] of the National Research Council at Evans Memorial Hospital, 65 East Newton Street, Boston." The *Times* provided only a general outline of the program of the Committee, however. "Disposition of the request," the article noted, "will be determined by policies adopted and frequently reviewed by the Committee on Chemo-therapy [*sic*]." "Much time," the newspaper added, "would be saved if doctors in charge of cases would get in touch directly with Dr. Keefer." By the end of September 1943, Keefer had become the central public figure in penicillin rationing—particularly since the *Times* had even publicized his address.[17]

Some patients, newspapers reported, did receive penicillin. Following a call to Chester Keefer from a teenager's surgeon and the Governor of Pennsylvania—who offered to fly to Boston to make the request personally—the *Pittsburgh Post-Gazzette* reported that the COC chairman had approved the patient's treatment. When the eager reporter contacted Keefer, he explained, "I want to tell this kid something if I can, Doctor. Can't you give me an idea when we're likely to get this penicillin?" Keefer offered a characteristically succint reply: the child would receive the drug within two or three days. Other reports also appeared before the American public. From Minneapolis, the *Sunday Tribune* announced that seven-year-old Lawrence Knowles had improved miraculously after his sulfonamide-resistant infection had responded to penicillin. In August 1943, a Washington, D.C. paper joined in the chorus: "Penicillin Saves Life of Virginia Girl at Johns Hopkins."[18]

Although it is difficult to measure the impact that these newspaper accounts had upon laypersons, they seem to have fueled an enormous public interest in the drug. As early as February 1943, a *Time* article attracted the attention of William F. Baird, who proposed a refrigerated crate that could preserve a perishable product (such as penicillin) for over a week. Several months later, Private E. L. Alexander, stationed at Camp Siebert, Alabama, told the National Research Council that a *Life* article about the drug had inspired him to suggest an alternative mode of producing penicillin (which he patriotically offered to the government).[19]

The media had inspired Baird and Alexander to assist the war effort, but for most individuals the popular press raised unrealistic hopes of a miracle cure—just as A. N. Richards had feared. One Brooklyn teenager, writing to Franklin Roosevelt on behalf of his ailing mother, explained, "When we first heard of penicilium [sic] in the paper, we wrote to the doctor who wrote about it in the newspaper, and his answer to us was that he could not do anything about it." Another civilian, writing to the President from Idaho, explained that his grandmother had recently sent him a newspaper clipping about obtaining penicillin for a desperately ill relative. One woman wrote in September 1943 that she had "read in the Reader's Digest of ... using penicillin for different diseases and for diseases of the eyes." She hoped to get the drug for her brother, who had been blind for three years. The woman told the President, "I wrote to you as I have read where you have helped others like him."[20]

One of the most poignant pleas came from a distraught patient in Columbus, Ohio's White Cross Hospital: "HEARTLESS AND CRUEL IS THE ADDED BURDEN OF THE SUFFERING I BEAR READING DAILY RELEASES IN THE NEWSPAPERS SINGING THE PRAISES OF THE NEW WONDER DRUG PENICILLIN." The drug, he lamented, had even

"CURED DISEASES IN CACTUS PLANTS." The distraught patient added that his chronic prostate infection remained untreated because of the inability "TO SECURE ENOUGH PENICILLIN FOR ONE SUFFERING HUMAN BEING. SURELY PUBLICITY AND PRAISE HAVE HAD THEIR INNINGS," he pleaded. "WHEN DOES HUMANITY BEGIN TO BENEFIT? I AM SO TIRED OF THIS MISERY AND PAIN [capitals in original]."[21]

The press, apparently unconcerned with the effect of their reports on the American public, soon realized that their stories had created a celebrity: Chester Keefer. Robert D. Potter, science editor for *The American Weekly*, wished to focus on Keefer's work as COC chairman. Preparing a story on the subject, he assured A. N. Richards, "I know you folks are doing a good job and I should like to explain some of the problems of your committee to the public." Potter did not want "to pry into any restricted information," but he thought his report might clarify for Americans "the problems which face men like Dr. Chester Keefer with penicillin." "As you are only too well aware with the public crying out for greater allotment of penicillin," Potter added a week later, "men like Dr. Keefer are on the spot. I want to try and get them off the spot and show what difficult decisions they have to make ... and why."[22]

Richards cautiously accepted Potter's proposal. "Having become somewhat allergic to popular articles on penicillin and their effects," he told the reporter, "I feel inclined to invite you to let me see what you propose to publish in the article to which you allude, despite the obvious friendly intention with which it is written." The record of the press up to that time, however, had given Richards sound reasons for his suspicions. Few journalists had shown such an eagerness to cooperate with either the CMR or the COC.[23]

Potter ignored Richards's conditions. *The American Weekly*'s headlines proclaimed, "Heartbreaking King Solomon Dilemmas of 'Judge' Keefer" and captioned a photograph of "little Patty Malone," "Saved From Death When 'Judge' Keefer Granted Her Penicillin, Little Patty Malone Recognizes Her Happy Parents for the

First Time in Weeks." Patients who did not receive the drug, the caption added, had acted as heroically as soldiers on the front.[24]

The *Weekly* reminded civilians that Chester Keefer was "the final authority in America" on civilian penicillin distribution. Suggesting that Keefer's guidelines represented "a new set of rules unlike anything in medical or judicial history," the spread's most dramatic caption challenged its readers to consider swapping roles with "the Allocator of Life-Saving Drugs Who Decides Whether a Soldier, Sailor, Civilian, Child, or Adult Must Face Death So That Others Can Live." Potter soberly described Keefer's office: "In front of you, on your desk, you have a complete history of the case, from the first diagnosis by the family physician up to the moment when an appeal was made to you." To complicate matters further, he continued, the COC chairman's desk was cluttered with petitions "from many people—begging you to decide in their favor, and telegrams from prominent personages who had been urged to intercede in her behalf."[25]

John G. Rogers of the *New York Herald Tribune* followed Potter's lead. Keefer, Rogers asserted, was "a one-man ration board." "Several hundred times a week," he wrote, "by letter, wire, or telephone, doctors or laymen from Maine to California ask Dr. Keefer for penicillin." The decision remained his alone, the report continued dramatically: "A baby is dying in Minnesota . . . a mother in Texas is losing her fight against a rare blood disease . . . an accident victim in Nebraska is failing to respond to all known treatment. Penicillin might help."[26]

While these journalists may have believed that they were helping the COC, Keefer believed newspaper reporters had undermined the efficient and equitable rationing of the drug. Keefer bristled at his popular notoriety. He had basked in professional repute but perceived news-hungry reporters as menaces who were only concerned with publishing sensationalized articles. Keefer told A. N. Richards, "I haven't always been successful in suppressing undesirable publicity." Journalists, Keefer added cynically, "tell everyone that they are concerned with saving lives and want to help. No one who has ever had any dealings with newspaper reporters should be naive enough to believe this story."[27]

Keefer also felt that these reports misrepresented his own work and the policy of his Committee. Although he was responsible for release of the drug to civilians, he based his decisions on the results of the clinical research of accredited investigators and the judgment of the Committee. Furthermore, Keefer resented the epithet "Judge" and assertions that he was a heartless bureaucrat, insensitive to the pleas of ill civilians. Sensational press releases about his role in the rationing program, he emphasized, were blatantly counterfactual. Keefer's contemporaries insist that he was an orderly and reticent individual, but he was no cold-hearted bureaucrat. He perceived his task as advancing clinical science and insuring equitable distribution of the drug. Referring to Marie Barker, a Chicago teenager who died of bacterial endocarditis in August 1943, Keefer wrote that the press had often made "misleading and incorrect" statements about her case and had painted him as cruel and stoic.[28]

Keefer offered A. N. Richards another example of newspaper mishandling of a penicillin request from Atlanta, Georgia. After receiving a call from the editor of the *Atlanta Constitution* at 11:15 p.m., Keefer explained that he could do nothing until morning. Three hours later an Atlanta physician telephoned to say that over a dozen journalists had already insisted that he contact Keefer. The beleaguered doctor acquiesced to their demands in order to satisfy the relentless reporters who had been hounding him. Keefer released the drug the next morning but warned the physician to make no statements to the press. Shortly after, however, the "United Press" phoned Keefer about rumors that the "material" had been released to an Atlanta doctor. "Where was it being shipped from? When would it come?" the caller queried, but Keefer refused to divulge any information.[29]

Keefer remained uncooperative when questioned by the Associated Press and International News Service, but additional details managed to leak to the press. The attending physician finally confessed to Keefer that he had tried to thwart the inquisitive reporters, but they had learned which flight was transporting the drug "and had the penicillin transferred from the mail compartment in care of the pilot." The press was waiting at the Atlanta airport, Keefer wrote, "took it in tow and approached Grady Hospital with the trumpets blaring."[30]

Reports of "home-made penicillin" also complicated penicillin rationing, since the media gave the dangerous impression that production of the drug was a relatively simple matter. *Science News Letter* reported in November 1943 that any doctor could produce in his kitchen "crude penicillin for [topical] treatment of staphylococcal and several other coccal infections." The article featured Dr. Julius Vogel, of Aliquippa, Pennsylvania, who had obtained a starter culture of *Penicillium notatum* from a hospital in Pittsburgh. Vogel reported promising results after treating twenty-nine patients. It was all very simple, he explained. Vogel had used only "the usual equipment found in the average family kitchen of today." The doctor, *Science News Letter* told its readers, operated a "$5 Penicillin Factory."[31]

The *New York Times-Herald* in late November 1943 offered the most elaborate instructions for home-made penicillin. The news daily ran a full-page story about its science editor, Wilson Scott, "Ready to Go" with his "$10 investment in equipment and ingredients for making penicillin." Scott outlined several basic steps for growing penicillin and explained that after four days the sterile gauze on which the culture grew had yielded the mold. At this point, he asserted that one could use the material on minor cuts and abrasions but cautioned that "the poultice should never be used until laboratory tests prove it has not been contaminated."[32]

The popular press appeared more willing to clarify these reports of home-grown penicillin than it had news about Keefer or the rationing program. The press reported researchers' warnings of the dangers of lay-produced penicillin. On Christmas Day 1943, a letter from Kenneth Raper and Robert Coghill, who both worked at the Northern Regional Research Laboratory in Peoria, Illinois, appeared in the *Journal of the American Medical Association*. "During recent weeks," they wrote, "a number of scientific articles and press releases have appeared indicating that the production of penicillin preparations suitable for external use is a comparatively simple matter that can be undertaken in laboratories possessing only limited facilities, or even in the kitchen." Raper and Coghill warned, "Statements to the effect that Penicillium notatum is the green or blue mold found on bread, cheese or other foods are quite misleading if, in fact, not actually dangerous." Laypersons without sophisticated laboratory equipment would be unable to process and refine the mold properly. The *Washington Post* echoed this sentiment by also reporting the hazards of kitchen-produced penicillin. *Science News Letter* added its own "Penicillin Warning": "Homemade chemical from mold may be dangerous to use for medicinal purposes." Without careful laboratory analysis, one could not distinguish a harmless from a dangerous product. Only in the case of home-made penicillin did the media attempt to present a balanced account of the new drug.[33]

Although Richards and Keefer seldom succeeded in controlling publicity about penicillin, they did prevent production of motion pictures about the drug. H. H. MacDonald of Bendix Pictures, for example, appealed to the CMR and COC for assistance in completing a film about penicillin. Specifically, he requested a "detailed outline" of the process of penicillin production and its clinical use. When Keefer's staff forwarded the letter to A. N. Richards, the CMR chairman told MacDonald that films, in the same manner as press coverage, complicated the work of both the COC and CMR. He wrote that the distribution of newsreels or documentaries "at the present time or in the predictable future" might threaten the war effort, and it would intensify "civilian demands" for the drug. Home-front requests, Richards and Keefer knew all too well, had far exceeded the available supplies of penicillin.[34]

Richards also refused an October 1943 film request from the Office of War Information (OWI). Alexander Eliot told the CMR chairman that his agency wished to inform friendly nations about penicillin. The new drug, the OWI believed, brimmed with propaganda potential. "The story of Penicillin," Eliot argued, represented "a remarkable example of scientific cooperation" between British,

American, and Canadian physicians, scientists, and engineers. The Office of War Information, he added, wanted to emphasize the coordination of Allied research efforts since the Axis had employed propaganda to discredit American and British cooperation. Eliot hoped to cultivate the same collaborative ethic during the postwar years.[35]

Eliot told Richards that the nation's allies must not feel that the United States had refused to share its penicillin. Snippets of information about the drug, he continued, had "already reached the populations in these areas through short wave radio broadcast and other media emanating from the United States, England, and Russia." Looking to the future, Eliot concluded, the United States would be required to explain "the difficulties of providing this drug for mass distribution." Honesty, Eliot seemed to suggest, would forestall any allegations of secrecy or hording of penicillin.[36]

Richards refused Eliot's proposal for the same reason that he resisted all other publicity requests and also because he feared that this film might start a wave of penicillin requests with international dimensions. As it was, the Roosevelt Administration had already received foreign requests for the drug. Dissatisfied, the OWI asked that the CMR chairman place the matter before the Office of the Surgeon General. That office, however, supported Richards's opinion that the international release of a film about penicillin would be "premature."[37]

The inability of the Office of War Information to secure the cooperation of the CMR was typical of its relationship with many wartime agencies. Despite the OWI's desire to report both battlefield and home-front news, Allan Winkler has noted, many offices (often for reasons of security) provided sketchy—if any—information, a source of frustration for the OWI. As surveys had shown, well-informed civilians were far more likely to support the war effort. The OWI Director, Elmer Davis, constantly tried to convince wartime agencies and the armed forces to give him information that his staff could "make intelligible." Although the Committee on Medical Research and War Production Board provided the OWI with periodic reports on penicillin, these releases included only brief information that followed security guidelines.[38]

The CMR and the COC also refused requests for radio broadcasts. Kathleen Goldsmith of the Office of War Information contacted Keefer in October 1943 about including news of penicillin in its worldwide shortwave programs. The OWI, she told him, was eager to air news of American scientific advances. As a convenience to Keefer, the agency even offered to record his talk in Boston, but he refused after consultation with A. N. Richards. Both men believed that such broadcasts were inadvisable at that time. Radio publicity held as much potential as films and press releases for increasing domestic and international requests for penicillin.[39]

Only cartoons, perhaps because of their light-hearted tone, escaped the indignation of A. N. Richards and Chester Keefer. Forwarding a comic strip to Richards, an amused Robert Coghill joked that penicillin had truly "reached the acme of public acclaim." "Lady Luck" in October 1943 foiled an Axis plot to steal a sample of the drug from the "Greenmold Laboratory." Introducing the plot of the strip, the heroine explained to one of the Greenmold janitors, "It's a new discovery. . A wonderful healing drug. . very scarce. . even the Army doesn't have nearly enough of it. . ." The enemy, the comic strip hinted, was well aware of this. Demanding thousands of dollars for a small vial of the drug, one of the spies' colleagues inquired, "I trust you two are aware of the value. . and scarcity of this Penicillin! The U.S. Army wants it bad!" Displaying a container of the drug, he exclaimed, "Looka that beautiful stuff!"[40]

Lady Luck outwitted the Nazi agent by substituting bathwater for the drug. Thanks to her cleverness, "Dr. Greenmold," the director of the laboratory, remarked, "The real Penicillin has been kept in the safe. . . . It was Lady Luck's idea to plant colored water in the test tubes to lure the criminals." She added with a grin, "I hate to think of his future when he delivers that bottle . . . to Berlin!"[41]

Several months later, Vannevar Bush sent A. N. Richards a *New Yorker* cartoon of a mother and her sad-eyed daughter leaving a movie theatre with *The Song of Bernadette*, a feature film released in the winter of 1943-1944 in which the main character died tragically, on the marquee. The mother explained to the bewildered child, "It all happened in the days before penicillin, you know, dear."[42]

Richards and Keefer showed much less concern over penicillin publicity throughout 1944 and 1945. Although the reasons for this remain unclear, it is likely the chairmen felt that increased supplies of penicillin permitted treatment of greater numbers of patients. Monthly production of the drug in the United States increased from .425 billion units in July 1943 to nearly 120 billion units a year later.[43]

The relative indifference of Chester Keefer and A. N. Richards to penicillin publicity throughout 1944 and 1945 could also be due to the changing character of media coverage of the drug. Commercial producers, eyeing lucrative postwar markets, began to advertise their role in the development of penicillin. Even companies that had shown little interest in penicillin rushed to place their products alongside the lifesaving drug. These ads stressed the central place of the drug in the postwar world, a message that meshed easily with the themes of other advertisements. Alongside futuristic copy that asked, "Will your Post-War House be a Soap Bubble?", "What wonders do you see in store for the Postwar Electrical Home?", or one, showing a vehicle—part-automobile, part-helicopter, and part-airplane—"What'll it be . . . wheels or wings?", advertisers couched the drug amidst descriptions of a postwar future unlike any ever before imagined.[44]

With a vial of "Penicillin-C.S.C." alongside a hypodermic syringe, an April 1944 Commercial Solvents Corporation advertisement reminded civilians of the central role the company had played in manufacturing the drug. The government, the ad noted proudly, had chosen Commercial Solvents to erect a plant that might soon be the world's leading penicillin producer. While the company's entire output remained under the control of the War Production Board, Commercial Solvents would, when military requirements had been met, lead the way in providing penicillin for all Americans.[45]

Another Commercial Solvents advertisement showed "Penicillin-C.S.C. in Production." Depicting its huge fermentation vats filled with thousands of gallons of penicillin culture, the chemical firm reminded the home front that "the medical profession is receiving larger quantities for the treatment of civilian patients." Taking a lighter tone, "Penicillin Is 'Shop Talk' to These Rabbits" depicted a researcher, hypodermic syringe in hand, testing the drug. According to a *Newsweek* article in summer 1944, the $1,750,000 Commercial Solvents plant utilized assembly lines "both for rabbits and wrappings" to package penicillin. The report reminded civilians that Commercial Solvents had helped to save "countless lives on the battlefront."[46]

Commercial Solvents presented its most poignant message to the American home front in *Newsweek*'s Christmas 1944 issue. Explaining "Why the Army Tells Us More of Our Boys Will Come Home!" the advertisement compared the mortality and morbidity from wounds and diseases of World War I and World War II. "In this war," the ad read, "97 out of every 100 wounded men recover—in sharp contrast to the 8% mortality in World War I." The advertisement reminded readers that Commercial Solvents Corporation had supplied large amounts of the penicillin that had saved many wounded servicemen.[47]

Other companies were also eager to associate their product with both penicillin and the war effort. Advertisements for everything from refrigerators to machine belts reminded Americans that even non-drug companies were involved—however marginally—in wartime penicillin production. One firm, Rusco Machine Belts, advertised in August 1944 that its products had been used in trucks that had rushed penicillin to the front. The ad concluded proudly, "Fortunate is RUSCO's destiny to be privileged to supply modern drug manufacturing laboratories with High-Speed Centrifuge Machine Belts which do their part in speeding the production of life-saving Penicillin."[48]

Another firm, York Refrigeration and Air Conditioning, emphasized that its role in penicillin production brought "new hope to the world of tomorrow." "In a great measure the triumph of penicillin is a triumph for air-conditioning and refrigeration," the copy noted. "At Cheplin, Hayden, Lederle, Pfizer and Reichel—mass producers of penicillin—York-built air conditioning systems keep the nurturing tanks at just the right temperature for proper growth." Worthington Air Conditioning added in June 1945, "Today, we're getting penicillin in the quantities we need, with the help of this better air conditioning." The advertisement also assured consumers that they too would "thrive in this 'culture medium.' "[49]

Electronics companies also linked their products with penicillin. Westinghouse, for example, stressed that its Mazda Lamps, which had provided "See-ability" for penicillin researchers, had played a crucial role in the production of the drug. "For in Penicillin culture," the ad stated, "technicians must measure and weigh minute quantities, compare sample compounds, detect infinitesimal color gradations . . . all vital close-seeing operations where See-ability means better concentration and faster, more accurate work." Another Westinghouse ad suggested that electronics insured penicillin's purity. The copy noted that laboratory "processing rooms must be kept free of air-borne dust and bacteria. Electronic equipment does the job most efficiently."[50]

Announcing "New RCA Penicillin Process Speeds Production!" an August 1944 ad in *Newsweek* stated that "a single RCA electronic installation can concentrate two billion Oxford units of Penicillin in 24 hours—enough to administer 100,000 individual doses." Having installed an RCA "electronic dehydrator of penicillin" in Squibb's New Brunswick, New Jersey, research facility, RCA added, "TODAY, when the wonder-drug penicillin is so vitally needed on the fighting fronts and in the home-front sickrooms, the Radio Corporation of America reveals that a revolutionary method of production has been perfected in RCA laboratories."[51] Even advertising firms themselves extolled the virtues of penicillin. In late 1944, for example, H. W. Ayer and Sons posed, "Why did penicillin almost perish?" According to the Ayer company, Americans had cast their sights too low, their dreams had not been bold enough. "There is no limit," the copy began, "to the possibilities for expansion and growth if we will open our minds to new ideas, and intelligently apply our new-found scientific knowledge, our inventiveness, our will to achieve." Postwar horizons seemed limitless.[52]

By the end of the war, penicillin had become generally available on the American home front, a fact emphasized by the Commercial Solvents Corporation. While one advertisement pictured a proud veterinarian and a heifer above the caption, "Cows need penicillin, too," another announced that "Penicillin has gone to the dogs." "Penicillin-C.S.C.," the advertisement read, "is now produced in such abundant quantities that it is available to veterinarians for treating farm livestock and domestic pets. Already it has saved the lives of many valuable animals." The ad concluded proudly, "Today Commercial Solvents is one of the world's largest producers of this life-saving substance."[53]

Champ Lyons found one of the advertisements humorous. Late in the war he sent one of his colleagues an ad that asked, "In this age of radar ... plastic magic ... and penicillin ... who is surprised at Biodyne R [a beauty cream]?" "This may not have your approval for burns," he joked, "but you sure missed a gold mine."[54]

Penicillin finally received wide attention in radio and film in 1944 and 1945. By that time, the drug had become much more generally available. In mid-June 1944, less than two weeks after medics had administered penicillin to D-Day casualties, the *National Farm and Home Hour* on the NBC Blue Network aired an entire program on "Penicillin Research at the Northern Regional [Research] Laboratory." The announcer began by telling his listeners that the broadcast would describe—as far as security restrictions would allow—penicillin production methods. Robert Coghill, an engineer at the laboratory who had been instrumental in developing fermentation technology for penicillin mass production, informed his listening audience that production was "increasing at a rapid rate and more penicillin is being allocated for civilian use every day ... in fact, 2100 hospitals now receive it."[55]

Keefer in one case personally endorsed publicity of penicillin. When Squibb proposed "an educational film on the use of penicillin" in March 1945, the same month that the drug went on sale through pharmacies, Keefer supported the idea. He told the War Production Board that the COC and CMR were vitally interested in the correct use of penicillin in medical practice. He believed that the film would prove invaluable in educating military and civilian physicians alike.[56]

Civilians also learned about penicillin from newsreels. Throughout the final year of the war this popular medium informed American moviegoers of the new drug. One lighthearted Paramount clip described a prize bull in Hardwick, Massachusetts, that received an injection of penicillin. Most newsreels, however, depicted the wonder drug in a more sober light. United News, for example, presented reports on penicillin production and the drug's use following the Normandy invasion.[57]

Few serious conflicts occurred during 1944 and 1945 between the media and the COC or CMR. However, occasional problems arose. John Fulton, a renowned Yale physiologist and personal friend of Howard Florey, contacted Chester Keefer in July 1944 about the appearance of Alexander Fleming's picture on the cover of *Time*. Florey, Fulton told Keefer, "seems to be utterly infuriated by the recent account of penicillin in *Time* and he hopes that we will exert our best efforts to avoid taking up a collection for the discoverers of penicillin." Fulton hoped that the National Research Council, Division of Medical Sciences, and Committee on Medical Research might give the public a "proper perspective" on "the most important medical discovery of our time." The continued notoriety of Fleming, however, suggests that the CMR and NRC had little influence on the press in this matter.[58]

On another occasion in October 1944, a Merck researcher overheard a radio announcer on the John Vandercook Program allude to a top-secret aspect of the penicillin program. Learning this, Hans T. Clarke, special assistant to the director of the Office of Scientific Research and Development, contacted Vandercook at New York City's WEAF. His office, Clarke informed the radio personality, was concerned about "public statements" on certain topics "officially classified as secret." Clarke underscored the point that his questions were prompted by reasons of national security not mere curiosity. While it is unclear whether Clarke ever located the culprit, Vandercook insisted that he had made "no reference to penicillin on any recent broadcast."[59]

Although Richards emphasized humanitarian concerns in his attempts to control publicity about penicillin, security restrictions may also have made him reticent about reports of the drug. From its inception, the CMR wished to "avoid publicity." Through "a code of quasi censorship rules" all information about penicillin was passed through the CMR before public dissemination. When the Washington Rotary Club asked Robert Coghill to give a talk on penicillin in late 1943, for example, he first sought Richards's approval. Even when production firms initiated advertisements about their role in production efforts, their copy skillfully avoided allusions to the chemistry of the drug or its production. Thus, security was maintained, and conflicts with the CMR and COC were avoided.[60]

It was the question of publicizing—and even sensationalizing—penicillin while supplies remained scarce that had placed Richards and Keefer at odds with the media. Faced with the relentless badgering of journalists (in addition to their own administrative responsibilities) Keefer and Richards could do little to silence their stories. Moreover, many newspapermen were unwilling to allow any governmental agency to quash the freedom of the press. Had the press censored itself, penicillin rationing would have been a far easier task for Keefer.[61]

On the other hand, the extensive reportage about wartime penicillin provided the lay public with an abundance of information on the drug. Furthermore, the news reports and advertisements about the drug had created a ready-made consumer market once the war had ended. Although the popular media seldom discussed the technical aspects of penicillin production, it presented undeniable evidence that the drug was effective yet relatively nontoxic. Long after "Judge" Keefer and A. N. Richards had faded from the public eye, the "wonder drug of 1943" remained firmly entrenched in the mind of the American public.

Notes

1. See especially Chester S. Keefer to A. N. Richards, 7 September 1943, Committee on Medical Research Files, Record Group 227, National Archives, Washington, D.C. [hereafter cited as CMR, RG 227]. See also David P. Adams, "Penicillin Mystique and the Popular Press (1935-1950)," *Pharmacy in History* 26 (1984): 134-142.

2. Chester S. Keefer to A. N. Richards, 18 December 1942, CMR, RG 227.

3. Jean Pinanski to A. N. Richards, 26 December 1942; E. C. Andrus to Jean Pinanski, 2 January 1943; A. N. Richards to Lawrence Dame, 4 December 1942; Catherine Coyne, "New Drug Passes Grove Fire Test," *Boston Herald*, 15 December 1942, clipping in CMR, RG 227.

4. Eleanor A. Bliss to E. Cowles Andrus, 30 November 1942; E. Cowles Andrus to Eleanor A. Bliss, 8 December 1942, CMR, RG 227.

5. John C. Sheehan, *The Enchanted Ring: The Untold Story of Penicillin* (Cambridge, Mass., 1982), 43; A. N. Richards to Edward Hutchings, Jr., 9 June 1943, CMR, RG 227.

6. See especially A. N. Richards, "Penicillin: Statement Released by Committee on Medical Research," *Journal of the American Medical Association* 122 (22 May 1943): 235-236.

7. A. N. Richards to Edward Hutchings, 9 June 1943, CMR, RG 227.

8. Allan M. Winkler, *The Politics of Propaganda: The Office of War Information, 1942-1945* (New Haven, 1978), 53.

9. "Penicillin Saves Child," *New York Times*, 26 September 1943, 28; "Penicillin Is Flown to Girl by the Army," *New York Times*, 5 September 1943, 31.

10. "Army to Get Its Magic Penicillin, Needs 5 Billion Units Weekly," *New York Herald-Tribune*, 30 July 1943, 1; Geo. [?] to A.N. Richards, 30 July 1943 [?], CMR, RG 227.

A "Rush on Penicillin" 125

11. " 'Wonder Drug' Pencillin [sic] Brings Magic Healing to Army," n. s., 16 June 1943; Irmis Johnson, "Penicillin: New Wonder Drug from Mold," *American Weekly*, 18 July 1943, clippings in CMR, RG 227; "Penicillin Use Honored," *New York Times*, 14 January 1944, 9.

12. Mona Gardner, "Miracle from Mold," *Woman's Home Companion*, September 1943, 70.

13. Paul R. Robinson to the Committee on Medical Research, 17 June 1943; see also Roger G. Prentiss, Jr., to A. N. Richards, 24 August 1943, CMR, RG 227; "More Penicillin," *New York Times*, 1 August 1943, sect. 4, 7. Despite the swelling public excitement about penicillin, no organized movement emerged to protest the COC rationing policy.

14. A. N. Richards to C. F. Speh, 31 July 1943; War Department, Surgeon General's Office Memorandum, "Subject: Penicillin," 20 August 1943, 2, CMR, RG 227.

15. A. N. Richards to Morris Fishbein, 31 July 1943; Chester S. Keefer to Eugene Worley, 13 September 1943, CMR, RG 227.

16. "Rush on Penicillin," *Time*, 30 August 1943, 44-46; "Public Vies with Army for Penicillin, Miracle Drug that Comes from Mold," *Newsweek*, 30 August 1943, 68.

17. "Penicillin Supply Is Far Short of Demand; Army Gets Less than Half, Says Gen. Kirk," *New York Times*, 28 August 1943, 24; "Set Plans to Rule Penicillin Supply," *New York Times*, 26 August 1943, 52.

18. "Penicillin Rushed Here to Give Youth Last Chance on Life," *Pittsburgh Post-Gazzette*, n. d.; "Penicillin Helps Save City Boy From Infection and Fever of 108," *Minneapolis Sunday Tribune*, n. d.; "Penicillin Saves Life of Virginia Girl at Johns Hopkins," [*Washington?*] *Times-Herald*, 17 August 1943, clippings in Penicillin File C39 (g), Kremer's Reference Files, University of Wisconsin-Madison, Madison, Wisconsin [hereafter cited as KRF].

19. William F. Baird to National Research Council, 11 February 1943; William F. Baird to Lewis H. Weed, 8 March 1943; Earl L. Alexander, Jr., to National War [sic] Research Council, 25 June 1943; E. H. Cushing to E. L. Alexander, 29 June 1943, Committees on Military Medicine Files, Committee on Chemotherapeutic and Other Agents, National Academy of Sciences, Washington, D.C. [Hereafter cited as COMM, NAS].

20. Jack Hunter to Franklin Roosevelt, 29 October 1943; Don Mewherty to Franklin Roosevelt, November 1943 [?]; Mrs. M. A. Higgins to Franklin Roosevelt, 19 September 1943, CMR, RG 227.

21. Edward Shapiro to A. N. Richards, 22 March 1944, CMR, RG 227.

22. Robert D. Potter to A. N. Richards, 1 September 1943; Robert D. Potter to A. N. Richards, 13 September 1943; A. N. Richards to Robert D. Potter, 18 September 1943, CMR, RG 227.

23. Robert D. Potter, "Heartbreaking King Solomon Dilemmas of 'Judge' Keefer," *The American Weekly*, 17 October 1943, clipping in CMR, RG 227.

24. *Ibid.*

25. *Ibid.*

26. John G. Rogers, "Boston Doctor Finds Penicillin Rationing Hard," *New York Herald Tribune*, 17 October 1943, clippings in KRF.

27. Chester S. Keefer to A. N. Richards, 7 September 1943, CMR, RG 227.

28. Personal interview with Donald G. Anderson, Magnolia Springs, Ala., 5 January 1985; personal interview with Harry F. Dowling, Cockeysville, Md., 2 May 1986; personal interview with Thomas Forbes, New Haven, Conn., 13 August 1986; Chester S. Keefer, "Memorandum on the Case of Marie Barker," August 1943 [?], CMR, RG 227.

29. Chester S. Keefer to A. N. Richards, 7 September 1943, CMR, RG 227.

30. *Ibid.*

31. "Penicillin for All," *Science News Letter* 27 November 1943, 350; "$5 Penicillin Factory," *Science News Letter*, 4 December 1943, 364-365. See also "Making Penicillin in Home Suggested," *New York Times*, 11 November 1943, 24.

32. Wilson L. Scott, "Penicillin: Miracle Drug Produced in Times-Herald Test," 28 November 1943, *New York Times-Herald*, clipping in CMR, RG 227.

33. Kenneth B. Raper and Robert D. Coghill, "'Home Made' Penicillin," *Journal of the American Medical Association* 123 (25 December 1943): 1135; "Home-Made Penicillin Dangerous, Says Drug's Creator," *Washington Post*, 6 January 1944, clipping in KRF; "Penicillin Warning," *Science News Letter*, 1 Jan-

uary 1944, 12; see also "Penicillin," *New York Times*, 19 December 1943, sect. 4, 9.

34. H. H. MacDonald to Chester S. Keefer, 9 September 1943; Chester S. Keefer to H. H. MacDonald, 14 September 1943, A. N. Richards to H. H. MacDonald, 18 September 1943, CMR, RG 227.

35. Alexander Eliot to A. N. Richards, 29 October 1943, CMR, RG 227.

36. *Ibid.*

37. A. N. Richards to James S. Simmons, 13 November 1943, CMR, RG 227.

38. Winkler, *The Politics of Propaganda*, 51-52; Elmer Davis, "The OWI Has a Job," *Public Opinion Quarterly* 7 (Spring 1943): 8.

39. Kathleen Goldsmith to Chester S. Keefer, 21 October 1943; Chester S. Keefer to A. N. Richards, 25 October 1943; see also Chester S. Keefer to Kathleen Goldsmith, 25 October 1943, CMR, RG 227.

40. RDC [Robert D. Coghill] to A. N. Richards, 5 October 1943; Klaus Nordling, "Lady Luck," *Chicago Sun-Times*, 3 October 1943, 10-11, clipping in CMR, RG 227.

41. Nordling, "Lady Luck," 12.

42. "It all happened in the days before penicillin, you know, dear," *The New Yorker*, 4 March 1944, 25, clipping in CMR, RG 227.

43. Gladys L. Hobby, *Penicillin: Meeting the Challenge* (New Haven, 1985), 196.

44. "What'll It Be . . . Wheels or Wings?" *Newsweek*, 3 April 1944, 49; "Will Your Post-War House Be a Soap-Bubble?" *Newsweek* 10 April 1944, 97; "What Wonders Do You See in Store for the Postwar Electrical Home?" *Newsweek*, 30 April 1944, 45. For discussions of wartime advertising, see especially Frank W. Fox, *Madison Avenue Goes to War: The Strange Military Career of American Advertising*, Charles E. Merrill Monograph Series in Humanities and Social Sciences, 1 (Provo, Utah, 1975); John Morton Blum, *V Was for Victory: Politics and Culture during World War II* (New York, 1976); Adams, "The Penicillin Mystique and the Popular Press," 138-139.

45. "Penicillin . . . Life Saver," *Newsweek*, 17 April 1944.

46. Adams, "The Penicillin Mystique and the Popular Press," 139; "Penicillin Is 'Shop Talk' to These Rabbits," *Newsweek*, 10 July 1944, 1; "Mass Magic," *Newsweek*, 24 April 1944, 62.

47. "Why the Army Tells Us More of Our Boys Will Come Home!" *Newsweek*, 25 December 1944.

48. Adams, "The Penicillin Mystique and the Popular Press," 139; "How Belts Help Speed the Supply of Precious Penicillin," *Newsweek*, 7 August 1944, 56.

49. "Powder of Life," *Newsweek*, 16 October 1944, 63; "You'll Thrive in This Culture Medium," *Newsweek*, 18 June 1945; see also "How Penicillin Is Dried with Frick Refrigeration," *Newsweek*, 11 December 1944, 112.

50. "Penicillin Culture . . . a Job for Unerring Eyes," *Newsweek*, 28 August 1944; "Penicillin's Purity is Guarded by Electronics," *Newsweek*, 28 August 1944, 46.

51. "New RCA Penicillin Process Speeds Production," *Newsweek*, 21 August 1944, 69.

52. "Why Did Penicillin Almost Perish?" *Newsweek*, 6 November 1944, 83.

53. "Cows Need Penicillin, too," *Newsweek*, 3 September 1945, 1; "Penicillin Has Gone to the Dogs," *Newsweek*, 9 July 1945.

54. Champ [Lyons] to John [?], March 1945 [?]; "In This Age of Radar . . . Plastic Magic . . . and Penicillin . . . Who Is Surprised at Biodyne R?" clipping in CMR, RG 227.

55. "Penicillin Research at the Northern Regional Research Laboratory," 14-15, radio script in KRF.

56. Chester S. Keefer to Priorities Department, War Production Board, 23 March 1945, CMR, RG 227.

57. *Paramount News*, 19 January 1944, v. 4, no. 41; "New Service Speeds Mail to U.S. Troops," *United News*, 1944; "Royalty Christens U.S. Bomber," *United News*, 1944, RG 108, National Archives, Washington, D.C.

58. J. F. Fulton to Chester S. Keefer, 7 July 1944, CMR, RG 227; "Dr. Alexander Fleming: His Penicillin Will Save More Lives than War Can Spend," *Time*, 15 May 1944, front cover; "20th Century Seer," *Time*, 15 May 1944, 61-68; see also Gwyn MacFarlane, *Alexander Fleming: The Man and the Myth* (Cambridge, Mass., 1984).

59. Hans T. Clarke to J. W. Vandercook, 9 October 1944; John W. Vandercook to Hans T. Clarke, CMR, RG 227.

60. Sheehan, *The Enchanted Ring*, 54-55.

61. Adams, "The Penicillin Mystique and the Popular Press (1935-1950)," 134-142. An excellent contemporary discussion of penicillin production appeared in Albert L. Elder and Lawrence A. Monroe, "Penicillin: Wartime Growing Pains of the Industry," *Chemical and Metallurgical Engineering* 51 (March 1944): 103-105.

Chapter Five

The Office of Civilian Penicillin Distribution

The War Production Board in May 1944 transferred the responsibility of civilian penicillin rationing from the COC to the Office of Civilian Penicillin Distribution (OCPD). The increase in penicillin production by late winter of 1944—more than doubling between March and April 1944 alone—required a reorganization of the distribution system; the COC no longer could ration efficiently the growing supply of penicillin available for civilians. Although the COC continued its program of clinical investigation, the OCPD assumed the primary responsibility to distribute the drug to homefront patients. Utilizing the COC's guidelines for penicillin use, physicians at the OCPD's "depot" hospitals continued the equitable distribution of the drug while also attempting to prevent its improper use. When penicillin became commercially available in mid-March 1945, however, many of the fears of wartime clinicians materialized: improper prescribing of the drug and an insidious penicillin blackmarket in occupied Europe appeared with an alarming suddenness.[1]

Two factors prior to the winter of 1943-1944 had limited the mass production of penicillin. Surface cultures of penicillin mold had required a myriad of shallow fermentation dishes, and researchers remained unable to grow penicillin in sufficient quantities to satisfy either military or civilian requirements for the drug. Complicating matters further, John C. Sheehan observed, the final product oftentimes was impure. Until scientists and engineers could perfect more efficient methods, penicillin production increased slowly. Low monthly output, combined with increased military needs by summer 1943, had reduced amounts available for the home front.[2]

The research of microbiologist Norman G. Heatley and mycologist Andrew J. Moyer at the U.S. Department of Agriculture's Northern Regional Research Laboratory (NRRL) helped to overcome production obstacles. They discovered that corn steep liquor, a by-product of corn starch manufacture, provided an ideal penicillin growth medium. Subsequent research at the NRRL demonstrated that penicillin could even be produced within the liquor itself, rather than by low-yield surface methods. Pharmaceutical firms, aware of potential profits from the drug and the military's interest in penicillin, used this process to push production to record levels by early 1944. As the Eli Lilly Company had written to A. N. Richards in November 1943, the firm stood prepared "to more promptly fulfill our obligations to the armed forces and the public." It should be noted, however, as Vannevar Bush told the War Production Board's Donald Nelson a month later, that American penicillin manufacturers also wanted to avoid "any actions by the Department of Justice under the anti-trust laws of the Federal Trade Commission Act."[3]

Production increases provided greater quantities of penicillin for civilian patients, far more than had previously been available to them. To consider the future of the civilian penicillin rationing program, Fred Stock, chief of the War Production Board's Drugs and Cosmetics Branch, organized the Task Committee on Civilian Distribution (TCCD), a group of governmental and industrial representatives. Penicillin rationing, the TCCD suggested, could continue under Chester Keefer. The chairman of the Committee on Chemotherapy refused, however, stressing that his office lacked adequate facilities and personnel to distribute an additional three to five billion units of the drug per month. Although he supported the transfer of civilian rationing to another agency, Keefer emphasized that penicillin should remain tightly controlled. Centralized administration alone, he believed, insured the drug's proper use and efficient distribution. Above all, Keefer reminded the TCCD that his primary responsibility remained the clinical investigation—not distribution—of penicillin. He, nevertheless, agreed to handle "hardship cases" during the first months following the transfer of rationing duties.[4]

Chester Keefer was probably eager to relinquish the responsibility of penicillin rationing to civilian patients. Laypersons and professionals alike had criticized him and labeled him the "penicillin czar" for his unyielding control of the drug. The press had portrayed him as a heartless bureaucrat, while some colleagues had disapproved of his unwillingness to permit free use of penicillin. These attacks had greatly complicated his role as COC chairman and prevented him from devoting his full attention to the clinical evaluation of penicillin.[5]

Keefer's unwillingness to continue the drug's distribution forced the Task Committee to consider other options. One of those was that penicillin might have "indefinite allocation through the armed forces," with a substantial amount reserved for eligible civilian cases. Once a surplus of ten to fifteen billion units became available, the Task Committee also proposed that drug companies might distribute penicillin to civilians "under a percentage-of-production allocation." The TCCD warned, however, that this idea did not allow "rigid control of civilian distribution" and might spark "black-market operations and indiscriminate use of penicillin." Careful regulation of the drug, the TCCD believed, would provide the most effective way to insure its judicious use.[6]

The most promising alternative involved distribution through hospitals. This plan retained centralized control of rationing (such as was the case under Chester Keefer) and provided an efficient means for distributing larger quantities to home-front patients. The proposed system, the Task Committee believed, also permitted the equitable provision of penicillin to civilians "in the largest number of strategically located areas consistent with the limited quantities available." This plan, the TCCD added, reserved penicillin for cases in which it was effective and helped to prevent its improper use. Thus, Robert Fichelis, director of the Chemicals, Drugs, and Health Supplies Division of the Office of Civilian Requirements, said that the plan allowed greater control of distribution to civilians according to the clinical guidelines established by the COC. "At this stage," he stressed, "use in physicians' offices should not be considered, and the drug should be restricted to hospital use." Fichelis, as much as Chester Keefer, wished to insure that practitioners treated only penicillin-sensitive illnesses.[7]

The hospital rationing plan benefitted physicians in particular. The system, for example, kept doctors informed through monthly reports of the amount of the drug available. Finally, practitioners—and patients alike—would be assured penicillin of the highest quality and potency. (Typically, the drug had a refrigerated shelf life of only three to six months.) The plan stressed, however, that all penicillin available for civilians should be rationed by a central authority in order to insure "orderly, rapid, and effective" distribution of the drug.[8]

The new plan also benefitted the Roosevelt administration. No longer would the federal government (which purchased penicillin for the COC through contracts with the Committee on Medical Research) bear the costs of distribution or of the drug itself (except for supplies necessary for COC). The report emphasized this point, since the drug was costing the Roosevelt administration $5 million annually. Furthermore, the OCPD would streamline penicillin rationing by serving "as a clearing house" for civilian requests. Image-conscious penicillin producers, some of which had already initiated aggressive advertising campaigns, were quick to emphasize that government agencies such as the OCPD could share responsibility for sudden reductions in civilian supplies in the event of a military emergency.[9]

Distribution through hospitals remained also in the best interest of civilians, the TCCD concluded in April 1944. Hospitals provided an equitable and efficient system that made penicillin available to "the greatest number" of qualified patients. Health care facilities, more easily than retail pharmacies, could facilitate access to the drug in the event of a military emergency. Hospitals also permitted adequate refrigeration of penicillin and solved the complex problem of its use. Due to the "rapid excretion" of the drug, which required a patient to receive injections every few hours, hospitals provided convenience for both patients and health care personnel.[10]

All U.S. "hospitals, sanitoria and related institutions" (over 6,600 in 1944) did not receive penicillin during the first phase of the TCCD's distribution program. The Task Committee selected instead the 1,054 hospitals approved by the American Medical Association for internships and residencies, a plan which included all forty-eight states (except Wyoming, Nevada, Idaho, New Mexico, and South Dakota where alternative facilities would be selected). "A small number of institutions could be deducted from this list," the Task Committee reasoned, "because the diseases treated by them would not require Penicillin to any significant extent." These facilities included homes for the aged, the "incurable," the mentally disturbed, and the mentally retarded as well as drug, alcohol, and tuberculosis sanitoria. General hospitals, the TCCD believed, represented the most ideal choices for its program. These institutions were properly equipped, well organized, and of adequate size. Furthermore, interns and residents could acquire first-hand experience in the proper use of penicillin. If these physicians-in-training had the opportunity to learn the correct clinical indications of the drug, policy makers hoped, they might apply their experiences to prudent postwar prescribing habits.[11]

The Task Committee also devised a hospital "distributional formula" where a facility could purchase each month "an amount of Penicillin equal to its number of beds, times 100,000 units." If a particular hospital had one hundred beds, then that institution could purchase ten million units of penicillin each month. The Committee concluded that its distribution system was "beyond reproach as a fair, equitable system" that insured the most efficient use of the limited supply of penicillin.[12]

The Task Committee attempted to provide the most equitable access to penicillin as possible. A random sample of fifty-five communities with depot hospitals revealed populations ranging from 1,775 persons (Roseau, Minnesota) to 1,504,277 inhabitants (Los Angeles, California). Each community had an average of two hospitals and a population of approximately 115,000 persons. Simple statistical tests suggest a close relationship between the population of communities and the number of depot hospitals located in them. The amount of penicillin available to these areas remained proportional to their population, so that the TCCD distribution system did not favor either urban or rural regions.[13]

Closer scrutiny, however, reveals a major flaw in the TCCD's distributional formula. The program provided penicillin to most civilians, but denied potentially eligible institutionalized patients easy access to the drug. This was not surprising as New Deal reform sentiments tended to wither under the exigencies of wartime. Since these facilities did not receive their own supply of penicillin, staff physicians were forced to try to obtain the drug from a designated depot hospital.[14]

The institutionalized elderly, especially those for whom the sulfonamides proved toxic, probably suffered the most under the TCCD plan. Ernst Boas, a pioneer in the field of gerontology, noted in 1941 that pneumonia in aged patients had a high mortality rate. This was especially true of pneumonias caused by sulfonamide-resistant organisms. Another study noted that even immunization did not significantly reduce the number of deaths. Although penicillin proved highly effective against pneumococcal, streptococcal, and staphylococcal pneumonia, the institutionalized elderly were denied ready access to the drug. One physician lamented in November 1943 that nursing home patients represented "the forgotten people" of the United States. Confined to convalescent facilities, they were far removed from mainstream society.[15]

The policy of the Task Committee also slighted the institutionalized mentally ill. These patients, a study of mental hospitals noted in early 1944, often suffered serious traumatic injuries which were susceptible to dangerous infections. Another report lamented the war's adverse effect on the overall level of institutional care of the mentally ill. "There is a danger," its authors wrote in late 1943, "that the standards of care of mental patients, built up over many years, may be impaired." Prior to "the present emergency and preoccupation with getting on with the war," another writer observed, "much remained to be done before the care received by the mentally ill... deserved the name of hospital care."[16]

Peter Tyor and Leland Bell noted in their study of the care of the mentally retarded in America that by the 1940s only the most profoundly retarded remained institutionalized. Care of these individuals during the Second World War, the authors commented, "continually deteriorated and at many places grim, oppressive conditions developed." As wartime America focused upon the immediate problems of defense, the needs of the mentally retarded were easily overlooked. It is, perhaps, not surprising that the Task Committee dismissed the plight of these individuals as well.[17]

The cost of penicillin therapy may have placed an extreme financial burden upon poor patients. Although many Americans enjoyed a higher standard of living during the war than they had in the 1930s, a significant portion of the population remained poverty-stricken. In 1944, for example, ten million workers (a fourth of which held manufacturing jobs) earned less than sixty cents per hour. Persons on a fixed income (such as social security recipients) and unskilled workers were also hard-hit by wartime inflation—which included the rising cost of hospital care. Late in the war, Senate hearings on wartime wages, education, and health noted that twenty million Americans lived a marginal existence which required "the utmost thrift" for economic survival. Given these circumstances, the cost of penicillin treatment—even when the price of the drug had dropped to under two dollars per 100,000 units by the middle of 1944—may have posed an undue burden on many families living in precarious financial straits.[18]

Nonetheless, rationing through health care facilities seemed to be the best choice. "Depot hospitals" served a two-fold purpose. They provided the drug for their own patients and advised institutions not designated as depot facilities where penicillin could be obtained. To insure the correct use of the drug, the OCPD distributed Keefer's clinical guidelines to all depot hospitals. This brochure informed attending physicians of the proper use of the drug and stressed that all doctors should use penicillin only according to specific instructions. In this manner, patients could receive the most benefit from the drug.[19]

The Task Committee also recommended that the Penicillin Industry Advisory Committee choose a *"Penicillin Control Administrator"* [italics in original] to assume Chester Keefer's responsibility of rationing the drug. Working from a central penicillin distribution office, the administrator could insure the equitable and efficient distribution of the drug to civilians. To guarantee impartiality in rationing penicillin from specific companies, the Task Committee also suggested the appointment of someone not employed by a penicillin producer, an individual who could devote his complete attention to the project (and insulate himself from pharmaceutical company pressures to use their penicillin rather than their competitor's). After consideration of several nominees, the Task Committee selected John N. McDonnell. His background in both pharmaceuticals and bacteriology, experience with the War Production Board's Chemicals Bureau, and his position as editor of *The American Professional Pharmacist* made him an excellent choice as the penicillin control administrator.[20]

The Task Committee established McDonnell's office in Chicago and provided him with qualified staff to assist in the distribution of penicillin. A midwestern office, run by a full-time administrator and his personnel, and an increased penicillin supply was a considerable improvement over the rationing system under Chester Keefer. The Midwest provided a far more central location than Keefer's Boston office. Hospitals in California and New York, for example, were roughly equidistant from the OCPD central office. The new facility even boasted a full complement of clerical workers. While Keefer usually had a staff of three, the OCPD employed over a half-dozen office workers.[21]

On May 2, 1944, McDonnell informed Fred Stock, chief of the War Production Board's Drugs and Cosmetics Branch, that the agency had acquired sufficient office space, equipment, and supplies. Installation of four telephone lines and swift delivery of "three complete sets of address stickers for 8,000 hospitals in each set" had also facilitated the processing of penicillin requests. The OCPD was ready for action.[22]

The OCPD distributed penicillin quickly and efficiently by answering telegram requests with telegrams, and each letter with a written reply on the same day. The Office handled emergency calls for the drug by telephone call or telegram, depending upon the urgency of the particular case. The OCPD sent depot facility rosters to all hospitals. The penicillin control administrator and Office of Civilian Penicillin Distribution informed all depot hospitals of their monthly penicillin allotment. A special bureau handled requests, approved "the order for sale," and determined which manufacturer would supply the penicillin. A daily "summary sheet" of all requisitions provided an ongoing record of monthly purchases of the drug. The OCPD required penicillin producers to ship all orders as promptly as possible, boasting: "Speed and accuracy the motto of this operation."[23]

McDonnell occasionally modified the TCCD's original distributional formula of 100,000 units of penicillin per bed per month, since fluctuating military requirements sometimes caused a reduction in the amount of the drug available for civilians. Manufacturers usually shipped the drug in ampules or vials of 100,000 units of sodium salt penicillin. Included would be detailed instructions by Chester Keefer, "Penicillin: The Indications, Contraindications, Mode of Administration and Dosage for Penicillin." These guidelines explained the necessity of the careful use of the drug and requested that all physicians follow Keefer's directions to the letter.[24]

The transfer of penicillin rationing to the OCPD attracted media attention, but McDonnell refused interviews by inquisitive reporters. Instead, he referred journalists to the Office of War Information. Articles had appeared in newspapers and trade journals, McDonnell wrote, however their authors had based their reports on OWI releases or "printed literature" available from the OCPD. Journalists, McDonnell commented, were highly complimentary of both the Office of Civilian Penicillin Distribution and the War Production Board.[25]

Hospitals quickly assumed their role in the program of the Office of Civilian Penicillin Distribution. During the first month of the OCPD's operation, facilities submitted an average of two hundred mail requests, forty telegrams, and twenty-five telephone calls daily. The number of petitions had escalated so markedly, the Office's May 1944 report stated, that all forty-eight states and the territories of Alaska and Puerto Rico had contacted McDonnell's office. Requests had even come from Canada. Health care facilities seemed to understand the new procedure especially well, and physicians and the public were pleased that penicillin had become available so "far ahead" of schedule.[26]

However, the system was not without its critics. Some hospitals, for example, objected to variations in the cost of penicillin; while the wide price differentials primarily affected the patients, the cost of keeping proper medication records and the variability of the cost of the drug remained a major inconvenience to health care facilities.[27]

Druggists also voiced their "dissatisfaction" with the OCPD program. Pharmacies, critics charged, were as "qualified" as hospitals to distribute penicillin, yet the OCPD's system "encouraged" health care facilities to perform this function. Several months later, a leading pharmacy journal warned that "intervention in the distribution of drugs by Federal and other agencies under War-time necessity" did not bode well for the future. Who could predict where the government might stop? the writer hinted. "Approved at present by all," the writer warned, hospital distribution of penicillin "interferes with the normal free democratic distribution system"—no doubt the free market. Hospitals, the pharmacists argued, had usurped the drugstore's traditional role of selling medicinals.[28]

McDonnell, in his role as editor of *The American Professional Pharmacist*, attempted to soothe the pharmacists' objections. Their patience, he counseled, was in the best interest of the war effort. Druggists "will wait patiently, knowing that this plan means lives saved now, and that the plan works for the ultimate benefit of all." "The profession," McDonnell concluded, "may feel confident that the civilian distribution of penicillin will be accomplished as efficiently, carefully and as equitably as possible under these present conditions." McDonnell predicted that the drug might even be available to retail pharmacies by the latter part of the summer.[29] "Urgent needs are being cared for," one writer noted, "but the prescription pharmacist, as usual, suffers. One guess as to its general release date is only about as good as another," *The American Professional Pharmacist* complained in August 1944.[30]

Other issues, however, overshadowed the protests of the pharmacists. One physician commented, "A much more thorny problem is the allocation of relatively small amounts of penicillin among hosts of patients and doctors who need, or at least think they need, this modern miracle of therapy." He added, "Fantastic amounts of pressure are now brought upon the few people who have any penicillin at their disposal, through every sort of medical pleas and exortations from relatives and influential laymen." To alleviate potential problems, the physician recommended, hospitals should form a committee that included a pathologist and heads of each of its clinical departments with the authority "to determine eligibility of patients for [treatment with] penicillin."[31]

The hospital penicillin committee, the author recommended, should base all treatment decisions on COC guidelines. Foremost, the committee should require "an accurate *bacteriologic* diagnosis [italics in original]." It was insufficient to say that a patient had pneumonia, since pneumococcal pneumonia responded well to penicillin while pneumonia caused by Friedlander's bacillus did not. Penicillin used improperly meant that sufficient supplies of the drug might be unavailable for more deserving cases. Although penicillin was effective against a broad spectrum of bacterial infections, hospitals should restrict use of the drug to susceptible organisms alone. The physician concluded that "control of some sort is the only alternative to a condition painfully close to anarchy."[32]

Hospital penicillin committees, it should be noted, differed somewhat from the institutional ethics committees that appeared several decades later in health care facilities. Modern boards typically have only the "potential" to influence clinical decision making, and their members often include social workers, the clergy, ethicists, and attorneys, as well as physicians. In making recommendations about the treatment of a patient, they often consider both subjective and objective criteria ranging from prognosis to potential quality of life and burden upon the family or society. Their role, however, is often only an advisory one. Hospital penicillin committees, on the other hand, had the authority to determine whether or not a patient received the drug. Their members, all physicians, stressed the paramount importance of clinical and laboratory data in selecting cases for treatment.[33]

Penicillin rationing through the nation's hospital system had gotten off to a good start. Overall, McDonnell reported that the first month of the OCPD's work had been "expedited in as efficient a manner as possible." "We believe," he wrote, "that the service rendered by this office to the Industry, the medical profession, to hospitals and to the public has been such that the War Production Board should be assured of satisfactory reaction and comment." McDonnell speculated again that ample supplies of penicillin would soon be available for general distribution. However, increased military requirements in late 1944 and recognition of the drug's value in a broader range of illnesses (such as bacterial endocarditis) forced the continued hospital distribution of penicillin.[34]

The OCPD program had expanded rapidly during 1944. There were originally 1,040 depot hospitals, but by early 1945 the number had nearly tripled; by the end of the OCPD's operation, the number of facilities had reached 6,611. Between May and December 1944, the number of civilian requisitions for penicillin had risen from 12.2 billion to 35.2 billion units. Between May 1944 and January 1945, the OCPD had released 168.2 billion units of the drug, and the agency anticipated that February 1945 civilian penicillin supplies alone would reach a record 130 billion units.[35]

Increased penicillin production raised the issue of providing the drug to the home front "through normal distribution channels." Fred Stock stated in late February that the War Production Board planned to transfer penicillin from the Office of Civilian Penicillin Distribution to pharmacies by March 15. The OCPD office, however, planned to maintain operations until distribution had been completely transferred to retail pharmacies and drug wholesalers.[36]

When the OCPD ceased official operations in April 1945, the agency had placed over thirty thousand orders with penicillin distributors and delivered over 2.5 million 100,000-unit vials of penicillin. At prices (to patients) from $2.40 to $10, the drug had yielded around $8 million in sales. It is likely that both producers and hospitals stood to make considerable profit from the sales of penicillin. If, as the Federal Trade Commission reported, the actual cost of the drug in January 1945 was only around one dollar, then initial profits may have reached the billions. These figures reflected the production increases which had permitted depot hospitals to treat far more civilians than under the clinical trials of the COC. By the time the OCPD curtailed its activities, the average daily number of depot hospital patients was over one million, with nearly two million beds in over 6,600 hospitals, including six in Alaska, one in Hawaii, eight in Puerto Rico, and one in the U.S. Virgin Islands.[37]

The *Journal of the American Pharmaceutical Association* in April 1945 welcomed the pharmacy's role in penicillin distribution. "In the future, as now," the *Journal* announced, "pharmacists in all branches of the profession will play an important part in making penicillin readily available in effective forms which will save the lives of those who would be doomed by otherwise fatal infections." Pharmacists believed that they too had a responsibility to insure the proper use of the drug. To this end, the editors of the *Journal* presented its April 1945 issue "as a reference handbook and guide" for the prudent distribution and use of penicillin. After their complaints of being slighted by the OCPD, the pharmacists had finally been appeased.[38]

The popular press also hailed the increased availability of penicillin. *Science News Letter* featured "Penicillin for Civilians On Sale at Drug Stores" in its March 17, 1945 issue and praised the enormous gains made by American pharmaceutical manufacturers. The popular science publication wrote, "You will be able to see and perhaps to buy the chemical but it will be put up in a form for hypodermic injection for your doctor to give you." The *News Letter* attributed the general availability of penicillin to the fine cooperation of the drug's manufacturers.[39]

The commercial release of penicillin, however, raised warnings about its injudicious use. *Science News Letter* and *Newsweek*, echoing the clinical guidelines of the Committee on Chemotherapy, reported that the drug effectively treated staphylococcal, streptococcal, and gonococcal infections. *Science News Letter* added that penicillin remained ineffective against polio, viral infections, and cancer. *Newsweek* cautioned that "the War Department [sic] . . . wants it understood that there is not enough [of the drug] to be wasted."[40]

Some of the gnawing concerns of the Task Committee materialized when penicillin became commercially available. No sooner had the drug emerged from "strict government control," John C. Sheehan wrote, than a thriving black market surfaced. "The first recorded attempt to export penicillin without a license—that is smuggle—was detected in the end of March 1945," Sheehan noted. The *New York Times* reported on March 31—scarcely two weeks after penicillin went on sale through commercial channels—that treasury agents had confiscated over twenty-five million units of the drug in Laredo, Texas, shortly before illegal traffickers tried to ship it out of the country. Other cases also occurred. Customs officials caught a Portuguese seaman in June 1945 as he tried to smuggle 200 vials of penicillin out of the United States. Another sailor tried to sell three hundred vials of the drug, worth around $25,000 on the Cuban black market.[41]

The most "vile" penicillin blackmarket appeared in occupied Europe—where only the military forces could legally obtain the drug. Allied intelligence agents, for example, uncovered a German scheme to substitute crushed atabrine (an antimalarial drug) in penicillin vials with a value of around $800 each. The narrator of Graham Greene's *The Third Man*, a novel about the underworld of postwar Austria, added that racketeers even diluted "the penicillin [solution] with coloured water, and, in the case of penicillin dust, with sand. I keep a small museum in one drawer in my desk," he said, displaying his collection of illicit penicillin vials. Numerous deaths resulted from the tainted drug, Greene's protagonist continued, but none so horrible as those of meningitis-struck children who received adulterated penicillin. "A number of children simply died, and a number went off their heads," he concluded grimly. "You can see them now in the mental ward."[42]

The illicit trafficking of the drug began rather harmlessly, as military orderlies sold it to Austrian physicians. One vial "would fetch anything up to seventy pounds." "You might say that this was a form of distribution—unfair distribution because it benefited only the rich patient," Greene's character commented, but the original distribution [to military bases only] could hardly have a claim to greater fairness." Soon, however, "the big men saw big money" in blackmarket penicillin—and the price soared as greedy kingpins scrambled for their share of profits.[43]

A British medical officer, stationed in occupied Germany from 1946 to 1948, confirmed the grim tenor of the early postwar years. The physician regularly treated venereal disease among the troops while pneumonia and meningitis ravaged German children. He "frequently" turned away "distraught parents," some of whom even presented "their dying child as proof of their desperate need."[44]

The easy accessibility of penicillin in the United States created its own share of problems. A 1945 editorial in the *New England Journal of Medicine*, for example, predicted that "indiscriminate use" of penicillin might cause postwar shortages of the drug. The prestigious *Journal* also complained that penicillin was used in large amounts and in "many conditions irrespective of any demonstrated beneficial effects." Not only did many physicians place "blind reliance" on penicillin, using the drug in conditions against which it was ineffective, but such "antibiotic abandon" boosted the number of resistant bacteria.[45]

The Office of Civilian Penicillin Distribution from May 1944 until March 1945 increased the availability of penicillin for American civilians. The planning of the Task Committee insured a program that would operate efficiently, maintain proper control over the clinical use of penicillin, and ration the drug equitably. The system denied, however, a significant—albeit often forgotten—segment of the population, the institutionalized elderly, mentally ill, and mentally retarded patients. Nonetheless, the distribution program of the OCPD (and the COC before it) succeeded at circumventing the tragic situation in occupied Germany and Austria.

The rationing system of the Office of Civilian Penicillin Distribution bore only a superficial resemblance to the distribution program of the Committee on Chemotherapy. Both controlled access to (and use of) the drug and utilized the basic clinical guidelines established by the COC. Their major difference lay, however, in the fact that the COC's primary responsibility remained one of investigation while the OCPD and its depot hospitals focused their efforts upon distribution. Chester Keefer was only too happy to relinquish his role as penicillin "czar."

The Office of Civilian Penicillin Distribution also served as a practical intermediate step in the wartime rationing of penicillin on the American home front. The increased production of the drug was too great to continue efficient distribution through the Committee, yet it remained insufficient to allow commercial sale. The OCPD and its depot hospitals represented a compromise between the highly restricted distribution under Keefer and the sale of penicillin on the open market. The OCPD's system also provided a model for postwar streptomycin rationing.

Both laypersons and physicians benefitted from the rationing program of the OCPD. Although penicillin was not readily available for institutionalized patients, most deserving patients had relatively easy access to the drug. Doctors (especially recently graduated interns and residents) also had excellent opportunties to gain valuable experience in the proper use of penicillin. These practitioners became some of the first (other than those who received the drug from the COC) to treat patients with penicillin.

By the close of 1945, however, the fears of the Task Committee on Civilian Distribution had materialized. The commercial sale of penicillin—and the relaxation of distributional controls on the drug—created ominous problems. While some entrepreneurs attempted to sell penicillin on the European black market, many physicians began to prescribe the drug improperly. The home front, one writer commented, had grown weary of wartime sacrifices and restrictions. He added. "The public (God bless its long suffering soul) will not only expect to have the things it has heard of. . . it will, in all probability, expect to be paid two-fold in luxury and convenience for things it gave up for the duration." So it would be with penicillin.[46]

Notes

1. Proposal of the Task Committee on Civilian Distribution, 6 April 1944, 1, Record Group 179, War Production Board Files, National Archives, Washington, D.C. [hereafter cited as WPB, RG 179].

2. John C. Sheehan, *The Enchanted Ring: The Untold Story of Penicillin* (Cambridge, Mass., 1982), 67.

3. *Ibid.*, 67-68; Gladys L. Hobby, *Penicillin: Meeting the Challenge* (New Haven, 1985), 87-110; Eli Lilly to A. N. Richards, 12 November 1943, Committee on Medical Research Files, Record Group 227, National Archives, Washington, D.C. [hereafter cited as CMR, RG 227]; Vannevar Bush to Donald M. Nelson, 4 December 1943, CMR, RG 227.

    The production contracts undertaken by American penicillin manufacturers came under close scrutiny by over a half dozen Justice Department lawyers to insure no violations of the Federal Trade Commission Act, designed to prevent a monopoly by a single company. See especially John T. Connor to Oscar Cox, 2 December 1943, CMR, RG 227; see also Peter H. Irons, *The New Deal Lawyers* (Princeton, N.J., 1982) for a discussion of the role of Justice Department attorneys during the Roosevelt era.

4. "Penicillin Producers Industry Advisory Committee, Summary of Meeting," 15 March 1944, 4, WPB, RG 179.

5. See especially Chester Keefer to A. N. Richards, 7 September 1943, CMR, RG 227.

6. "Penicillin Producers Industry Advisory Committee, Summary of Meeting", 15 March 1944, 4, WPB, RG 179.

7. Proposal of the Task Committee on Civilian Distribution, 6 April 1944, 1, 8, WPB, RG 179.

8. *Ibid.*, 8.

9. *Ibid.*; Hobby, *Penicillin: Meeting the Challenge*, 186-187.

10. *Ibid.*, 1.

11. *Ibid.*, 2-4.

12. *Ibid.*, 5-6. If *every* patient in a given depot hospital suffered from a penicillin-sensitive condition, then the allocation of 100,000 units per bed may not have been sufficient. Typical staphylococcic infections, for example, sometimes required more than a week of treatment with dosages in excess of 100,000 units per day. One may safely assume, however, that all patients did not require the drug.

13. The sample upon which the analysis was based included every tenth community (n=55) listed in War Production Board Press Release 5617, 4 May 1944, Office of War Information Files, Record Group 208, National Archives Annex, Suitland, Md. The statistical test, Pearson product-moment correlation coefficient, was employed. Comparison of the number of depot hospitals with the population of their communities yielded an extremely high value (r=.87), suggesting a highly significant statistical relationship (p< .05).

14. Proposal of the Task Committee on Civilian Distribution, 6 April 1944, 7, WPB, RG 179.

15. Ernst P. Boas, *Treatment of the Patient Past Fifty* (Chicago, 1941), 269-273; Paul Kaufman, "Prophylactic Effect of Pneumococcus Polysaccharide Against Pneumonia," *Archives of Internal Medicine* 61 (1941): 304-319; Paul Kaufman, "Effect and Toxic Effect of Sulfapyridine in Old Age Pneumonia," *New York State Journal of Medicine* 40 (1940): 204-208; Frederick W. Filsinger, "The Forgotten People," *Hospital Management* 56 (November 1943): 20-21.

16. Walter W. Jetter and Rollin V. Hadley, "A Study of Casualties in Institutions under the Supervision of the Massachusetts Department of Health," *American Journal of Psychiatry* 100 (January 1944): 515; Robert Woodman, "There Is Room for Improvement in Our Mental Disease Hospitals: Facts and Figures on These Public Hospitals—What to Do About Them," *Modern Hospital* 61 (November 1943): 78. See also Oscar Felsenfeld, "Yeast-like Fungi in the Intestinal Tract of Chronically Institutionalized Patients," *American Journal of Medical Science* 207 (January 1944): 60-62.

17. Peter L. Tyor and Leland V. Bell, *Caring for the Retarded in America: A History*, Contributions in Medical History, no. 15 (Westport, Conn., 1984), 137.

18. Cited in Richard Polenberg, *War and Society in the United States: 1941-1945* (New York, 1972), 87-88; "Cost of Living in Large Cities, April 15, 1943," *Monthly Labor Review* 61 (August 1945): 1178-1179.

19. Proposal of the Task Committee on Civilian Distribution, 6 April 1944, 7; [Chester S. Keefer], "Penicillin: The Indications, Contraindications, Mode of Administration and Dosage for Penicillin," n.d., 7, WPB, RG 179.

20. Proposal of the Task Committee on Civilian Distribution, 6 April 1944, 5, WPB, RG 179.

21. *Ibid.*; personal interview with Constance Haynes MacDonald, 29 May 1985, Boston, Mass.

22. John N. McDonnell to Fred J. Stock, 2 May 1944; "Report of the Office of Civilian Penicillin Distribution: Month of May, 1944," 9, WPB, RG 179.

23. Proposal of the Task Committee on Civilian Distribution, 6 April 1944, 6-7, WPB, RG 179.

24. "Distribution Procedure for Penicillin to Civilians," 1 May 1944, 1-4; [Keefer], "Penicillin: The Indications, Contraindications, Mode of Administration and Dosage for Penicillin," no date, 7, WPB, RG 179.

25. "Report of the Office of Civilian Penicillin Distribution: Month of May, 1944," 9, WPB, RG 179.

26. *Ibid.*, 6-8; John N. McDonnell to Fred J. Stock, 2 May 1944, WPB, RG 179.

27. "Report of the Office of Civilian Penicillin Distribution: Month of May, 1944," 9, WPB, RG 179.

28. "Report of the Office of Civilian Penicillin Distribution: Month of May, 1944," 9-10, WPB, RG 179; [John N. McDonnell?], "What of the Morrow?" *American Professional Pharmacist* 10 (September 1944): 619, 653.

29. [John N. McDonnell?], "Penicillin," *American Professional Pharmacist* 10 (May 1944): 315.

30. [Editorial], "Penicillin," *American Professional Pharmacist* 10 (July 1944): 465; [Editorial], "Penicillin Sodium," *American Professional Pharmacist* 10 (August 1944): 539.

31. Paul M. Hamilton, "Some Points on the Control of Penicillin When It Is Sent to Hospitals," *Hospitals* 18 (May 1944): 62; see also "Penicillin for Civilians Ready Soon; Plan Distribution through Hospitals," *Hospitals* 18 (May 1944): 82.

32. *Ibid.* The term "Friedlander's Bacillus" was a contemporary designation for *Klebsiella pneumoniae.*

33. Ronald E. Cranford and A. Edward Doudera, "The Emergence of Institutional Ethics Committees," *Law, Medicine, and Health Care* (February 1984): 13-20; see also John A. Robertson, "Committees as Decision Makers: Alternative Structures and Responsibilities," in Ronald E. Cranford and A. Edward Doudera, eds., *Institutional Ethics Committees and Health Care Decision Making* (Ann Arbor, Mich., 1984), 85-86.

34. "Report of the Office of Civilian Penicillin Distribution: Month of July, 1944," 1,; "Report of the Civilian Penicillin Distribution Unit (Office of Civilian Penicillin Distribution): Month of September 1944," 1, WPB, RG 179.

35. War Production Board, Office of Industry Advisory Committees, Summary of Meeting, 20 April 1945, 9; "Report of the Operations, from April 1944 to April 1945, inclusive, of the Office of Civilian Penicillin Distribution (Civilian Penicillin Distribution Unit)," RG 179, WPB.

36. War Production Board, Office of Industry Advisory Committees, Summary of Meeting, 30 January 1945, 10, WPB, RG 179; Hobby, *Penicillin: Meeting the Challenge*, 186-187.

37. "Report of the Operations, from April 1944 to April 1945, inclusive, of the Office of Civilian Penicillin Distribution (Civilian Penicillin Distribution Unit)," 5; "Depot Hospitals," 1 December 1944, WPB, RG 179.

38. "Penicillin Comes to the Corner Pharmacy," *Journal of the American Pharmaceutical Association* 6 (April 1945): 90; see also Robert P. Fichelis, "Penicillin: Opportunity and Obligation," *Journal of the American Pharmaceutical Association* 6 (April 1945): 91-92.

39. "Penicillin for Civilians On Sale at Drug Stores," *Science News Letter*, 17 March 1945, 168.

40. "Don't Waste Penicillin," *Science News Letter*, 24 March 1945, 179; "Ten for Penicillin," *Newsweek*, 26 March 1945, 93.

41. Sheehan, *The Enchanted Ring: The Untold Story of Penicillin*, 78; Patricia Spain Ward, "Antibiotics and International Relations at the Close of World War II," in John Parascandola, ed., *The History of Antibiotics: A Symposium* (Madison, Wis., 1980), 101-102.

42. *Ibid.*; Graham Greene, *The Third Man and the Fallen Idol* (London, 1964), 95-97.

43. *Ibid.*

44. C. V. Hey, letter to the editor, *British Medical Journal* (28 September 1974): 805; Lawrence P. Garrod, letter to the editor, *British Medical Journal* (28 September 1974): 805; see also Terry Hamblin, "Personal View," *British Medical Journal* (10 August 1974): 407.

45. "Abuse of Penicillin," *The New England Journal of Medicine* 233 (27 December 1945): 831; James C. Whorton, " 'Antibiotic Abandon': The Resurgence of Therapeutic Rationalism," in Parascandola, ed., *The History of Antibiotics*, 129.

46. Henry Welch and Felix Marti-Ibanez, *The Antibiotic Saga* (New York, 1960), 38; Donald Dailey, "What Will the Postwar Consumer Want?" *Advertising and Selling*, June 1943, 54. The problem of the overprescription of penicillin will be addressed in Chapter 6.

Chapter Six

The Legacy of Wartime Penicillin Rationing

The introduction of penicillin altered postwar medical practice and lay perceptions of physicians and drug therapy. Widespread beliefs about the panacean qualities of antimicrobial drugs influenced physicians' use—and abuse—of antibiotics. Amid a postwar "spree" of "antibiotic abandon" as pharmaceutical companies developed new drugs of this type, doctors spurned the clinical rigor championed by the COC. The academic medical community railed against the indiscriminate (and potentially dangerous) use of penicillin and other antibiotics, yet practitioners often ignored these warnings. Only after the overprescription of these drugs had reached alarming proportions did practicing physicians begin a return to the therapeutic prudence of the COC.[1]

The wartime penicillin program also accelerated the integration of academics into prominent policy-making positions. Since the Second World War, the State has relied increasingly upon the expertise of scientists and physicians to advise and direct scientific and medical policy. The penicillin project, an integral part of the American scientific and medical research effort, also demonstrated the ability of a well-funded research establishment to serve the United States in war and peace.[2]

In addition, penicillin rationing provided Americans with a foretaste of the distributional issues that were to become more critical in the decades ahead. By 1946, the COC applied its wartime experience to a new drug, streptomycin. As medical technology and drug therapy expanded during the postwar years, AZT, donor organs, and dialysis machines replaced antibiotics as the scarce medical resources of the late twentieth century.[3]

The increased availability of penicillin after March 1945 created an unexpected problem. Penicillin-resistant staphylococci, for example, quickly became a particular concern as penicillin became a mainstay of postwar drug therapy. One study found that while only 12.5 percent of the staphylococci cultured from patients in 1946 showed penicillin-resistance, the number had tripled by 1947 and had reached nearly 60 percent by 1948. One hospital had boasted only a 28 percent mortality rate for staphylococcal bacteremia in 1945, but in less than ten years it reached 80 percent—a level as high as the pre-penicillin era. "It became apparent," one researcher recalled, "that wherever penicillin was widely used, especially in hospitals, epidemics due to resistant staphylococci could break out." The *American Journal of Clinical Pathology* concluded that the typing of organisms for sensitivity determination represented "the keystone of planned penicillin therapy." Penicillin-resistant bacteria, many medical researchers feared, might one day render the drug ineffective.[4]

Donald Anderson and Chester Keefer raised the issue of penicillin-resistant bacteria in their 1948 monograph, *The Therapeutic Value of Penicillin*. In a number of unsuccessful cases, they wrote, physicians ascribed the drug's failure to penicillin-resistant staphylococci. Available data, they added, suggested that over 20 percent of staphylococcal infections "may develop" resistance to the drug. This phenomenon, Anderson and Keefer cautioned, "may constitute an important limitation to the successful use of the drug."[5]

Wartime researchers discovered other problems. Preliminary research published in the *Journal of Pharmacology and Experimental Therapeutics* and the *American Journal of Medical Science* in 1943 had suggested penicillin's potential toxicity, and Champ Lyons's studies in the spring and summer of that year confirmed these suspicions. After reviewing several of Lyons's cases, Chester Keefer told A. N. Richards that penicillin had caused several "problems." "First," Keefer reported, "a number of the patients have developed occlusion of their arm veins from the repeated injections of concentrated penicillin." Lyons, Keefer explained, hoped that more dilute solutions might alleviate the problem.[6]

Other problems included a small percentage of patients developing penicillin allergies. Lyons reported that penicillin had caused a " 'flushing' reaction" in some of his patients. Impurities in the drug, Lyons believed, caused this phenomenon, one that he thought careful filtration could rectify. Keefer speculated that the reaction posed no danger to the patient, but he felt that the COC should alert its investigators to the drug's potential side effects. And although the supplies sent by Squibb, Winthrop, and Pfizer later proved "painful on intramuscular injection," Lyons noted in late August 1943 that clinicians remained enthusiastic about penicillin. The drug, investigators agreed, had yielded "extremely impressive" results.[7]

No fatal reactions had occurred up to that time, and minor skin reactions remained insignificant in light of penicillin's ability to stem a raging infection. The alternative for a badly injured soldier or civilian child suffering from staphylococcal bacteremia might well have been disfigurement or death. Anderson and Keefer commented in 1948 that "amputation . . . was frequently obviated by the rapidity with which penicillin stopped the spread of the infection and effected healing of the local tissues." One D-Day casualty, for example, continued to receive penicillin injections despite the appearance of a generalized urticarial reaction on his torso and extremities.[8]

By mid-1945 a growing body of evidence confirmed the possibility of reactions to penicillin. The Food and Drug Administration's Adolph Rostenberg, Jr., and Henry Welch reported in 1945, "It would appear from the results of this investigation that a small, but substantial, percentage of the population" had a pre-existing sensitivity to penicillin. Chester Keefer agreed that same year that numerous researchers had observed allergic reactions, but he remained relatively unconcerned about the drug's toxicity.[9]

The Food and Drug Administration believed that impurities caused penicillin's toxicity. As a result, this same low-keyed attitude toward the drug's dangers also permeated Congressional hearings to guarantee the purity of "penicillin and derivative drugs." Certification of penicillin batches came as an amendment to the Food, Drug, and Cosmetic Act of 1938, endorsed by all who testified at the certification hearings. H.R. 3266, enacted in 1945, concerned itself with the certification of all "drugs composed wholly or partly of any kind of penicillin or any derivative thereof." This amendment was concerned only with penicillin's purity not its toxicity, since clinicians had tended to blame adverse reactions on impurities in the drug.[10]

One of the first summaries of penicillin reactions appeared in *The Therapeutic Value of Penicillin*, published in 1948. Donald Anderson and Chester Keefer listed sixteen types, from pain at the injection site to peripheral nerve damage. Nonetheless, only about 8 percent of patients had displayed allergies. Moreover, with the exception of one death (unrelated to the drug), Anderson and Keefer remarked that penicillin still had caused "no fatal reactions." They concluded in 1948 that relatively low toxicity made penicillin one of "the most remarkable of all the chemotherapeutic agents."[11]

That same year the *Annals of Allergy* published "Reactions to Penicillin: A Review of the Literature, 1943-1948." This survey of over three hundred articles confirmed the sensitizing effect of penicillin on some patients. *The Penicillin Decade*, published three years later, presented a more ominous message. The authors hoped that "surely the greater number of reactions recorded in these pages need not be found in penicillin's second decade." They concluded that the drug's "ability to sensitize and to cause serious and even fatal reactions should not be minimized. A grave responsibility rests upon the shoulders of the physician for its wise application in clinical practice." The message had become clear: penicillin could cause dangerous reactions in patients who were allergic to the drug.[12]

The burgeoning literature on bacterial resistance and allergy to penicillin, however, had little effect on the drug's postwar overprescription. The *Journal of the American Medical Association*, concerned about the overuse of the drug, cautioned in 1945 that the "penicillinization of our population" appeared imminent. The therapeutic value of penicillin had so overshadowed its potential shortcomings that some physicians feared that "penicillin might become the bacon and eggs of modern therapy." Raising these warnings in March 1945, even prior to the drug's general distribution, Dr. Leslie Falk submitted letters to the *Journal of the American Medical Association* and the *Journal of the American Pharmaceutical Association* in which he advocated "immediate measures" to stem the injudicious use of penicillin. He recommended, for example, additional research on penicillin toxicity and "adequate education of the doctor, the druggist, and the public . . . to assure the proper use (and restraint from use) of penicillin." James Whorton added, "Medical writers' uninhibited employment of the words 'miracle' and 'wonder,' and of proclamations such as 'a new era in medicine has begun,' were not calculated to promote careful prescribing."[13]

By the close of 1945, medical observers had characterized the prescription of penicillin as "a 'spree.'" The *New England Journal of Medicine* noted that many physicians prescribed penicillin for all febrile patients—and even those who *might* develop a fever or infection—whether or not the drug could alter the course of the illness. "Still more unsettling," Whorton observed, "were the cases of several physicians who knew themselves to have allergic tendencies, yet treated their own colds with penicillin—and died from the reaction." Even Alexander Fleming dosed his own viral respiratory infection with penicillin shortly before he received the Nobel Prize.[14]

The glowing reports about penicillin influenced practitioners' imprudent use of the drug. (In 1945, for example, the *Journal of the American Medical Association*'s readers voted penicillin as "the most valuable drug now used by the medical profession.")[15] Empirical evidence that an infection was treated successfully (or at least appeared to have been treated successfully), combined with the weight of opinion among local medical practitioners may also have contributed to the overprescription of antibiotics. Physicians in a given community, for example, often ignored the clinical rigor of their academic counterparts. Their busy office practices did not permit the time-consuming bacteriological tests demanded by Keefer and the COC. Moreover, one author noted, some practitioners failed to keep current with new indications for the drug; others were simply unable to understand the latest findings.[16]

Pharmaceutical company "detail men" (who market and promote new drugs to physicians) may also have influenced the overprescription of antibiotics. These salesmen showered doctors with "gifts and 'reminder items'" emblazoned with the drug name. In exchange for promotional items, practitioners may have felt obligated to reciprocate by prescribing the company's drugs. "When he cannot or will not do this," one observer concluded, "he feels guilty and may even *apologize* to the detail man [italics in original]."[17]

While a combination of professional and marketing pressures may have influenced physicians' injudicious prescription of antibiotics, patients probably played their own critical role. Historian of medicine Richard Shryock remarked that the outstanding results of antimicrobial drugs exerted an important effect on patients' attitudes toward the physician's ability to cure disease. Armed with panacean "miracle drugs," Harry Dowling added, postwar practitioners seemed capable of curing "just about everything." "So much had been discovered; people could not conceive that so much was still unknown," he concluded. Believing in penicillin's panacean powers, worried parents might have insisted that the physician at least *try* penicillin on their ill child—whether or not the drug was clinically indicated. When the illness improved, the layperson might have assumed that the penicillin had effected its course. Pressure of this type may well have convinced the physician, in the interest of calming the parent—or keeping the child as a patient—to acquiesce to the request. Moreover, these children may well have grown up with a mental image of antibiotics as panaceas and pressured their own children's physician to prescribe one of these drugs.[18]

The inability of some practitioners to heed—or even understand—the admonitions of academic physicians and resist patient pressure had made "the penicillin prescription" an expected part of

The Legacy of Wartime Penicillin Rationing 159

the visit to the doctor. Entrenched in American culture, the drug had become an icon of modern medicine. Even young children skipped rope to a penicillin-praising jingle:

> Mother, mother, I am ill!
> Call the doctor from over the hill!
> In came the doctor, in came the nurse,
> In came the lady with the alligator purse.
> Penicillin, said the doctor,
> Penicillin, said the nurse,
> Penicillin, said the lady with the alligator purse.[19]

Popular media coverage of penicillin also endowed the drug with curative powers that seemed to surpass those of the sulfonamides. Although the wartime press had reminded laypersons that the sulfas could "injure vital organs" and were toxic to millions of people, newspapers and advertisements portrayed penicillin in a much more benign light. The media ignored evidence in the professional literature of allergic reactions and penicillin-resistant organisms. The glowing popular reportage of penicillin, one study commented, consistently depicted a panacean drug that produced miracle cures without harmful side effects. In early 1945 *Time* even quipped that a combination of penicillin and streptomycin (one of the first post-penicillin antibiotics), "penicillin streptomycinate," might make clinical diagnosis unnecessary. Physicians, the article suggested, could use the drug "for all infectious diseases, and many of the courses in medical school could be abolished." At the end of 1945, for example, "use of the drug, streptomycin" ranked third in a *Time* list of the year's top ten scientific discoveries. *Reader's Digest* added that penicillin had conquered bacterial endocarditis, while a popular women's magazine announced the effectiveness of the drug against syphilis. One popular medical writer speculated that medical science, "as though propelled by destiny," would one day allow humankind "*to live in a world without menacing microbes* [italics in original]."[20]

J. D. Ratcliff, a contemporary medical writer, made one of the most impassioned pitches for penicillin in his 1945 *Yellow Magic:*

The Story of Penicillin. In addition to the usefulness of the drug against deadly diseases, penicillin would also have household uses, he predicted. "Dispensed as a salve, it would be valuable as a treatment for burns, cuts, and minor skin infections," Ratcliff remarked. "It might be sold in fluid form to be used as an eyewash, a nasal douche, a mouth wash to suppress trench mouth. It might even be added to contraceptive jellies to eliminate the possibility of venereal infection."[21]

Veterinarians and dentists, Ratcliff predicted, would also rely on penicillin. "From preliminary evidence it looks as if penicillin will be of great value in controlling barnyard diseases," he noted. The drug would also aid dentistry, Ratcliff continued. "Used in tooth-socket packing after extractions, penicillin should control the bacteria that frequently cause angry reactions." Penicillin-laden toothpaste, Alexander Fleming had predicted a year earlier, could treat diseases of the mouth and throat, many of which were caused by penicillin-sensitive bacteria. This product, the famed researcher intoned, would undoubtedly be used by persons suffering from minor oral infections.[22]

Penicillin lozenges, an early 1945 report announced, were also on the horizon to treat "strep throat." While the troches had a "very slightly bitter taste," they were easy to use when placed "in the cheek and left there to dissolve without sucking or chewing." They even appeared to be non-toxic: "One patient by mistake ate 10 of them during the first five minutes of treatment" without any ill effects. The writer seemed to suggest that penicillin was not very different from candy.[23]

Penicillin seemed to symbolize postwar medical and scientific progress. Reflecting upon 1945 America, historian Eric F. Goldman noted, "In a period when medical research had just produced the yellow magic of penicillin only to have it promptly topped by streptomycin, it did not seem utopian to talk of even conquering tuberculosis, infantile paralysis, even cancer." Moreover, Americans "could fill their gasoline tanks, use a second chunk of butter, watch the long lazy curl of a fishing line flicker in the sunlight, or get royally tight, without feeling that they were cheating some GI in the flak over Berlin or on the bloody ash of Iwo Jima." As penicillin became widely available in March 1945, civilian patients demanded the drug—and physicians could yield to their demands—without fear of denying it to a wounded soldier. At the same time, ironically, children in occupied Germany died for want of penicillin.[24]

Popular accounts of penicillin's dangers did not receive wide media attention until late summer 1949. *Consumer Reports* noted that as many as 10 percent of the patients who received penicillin experienced allergic reactions such as urticaria. Although most side effects were mild, "severe reactions" (such as anaphylactic shock) required "vigorous treatment measures." The periodical failed, however, to specify the precise nature of the "vigorous treatment measures."[25]

Coronet magazine elaborated in November 1949 upon the *Consumer Reports* article. The general interest monthly reported the death of a woman in 1948 from anaphylactic shock following an injection of penicillin. Shortly after her physician administered the drug, "the woman complained of a strange taste in her mouth, followed by swelling of the nose and throat. While leaning over a kitchen table," *Coronet* concluded gravely, "she suddenly collapsed. A few minutes later she was dead."[26]

This grim story had little effect on the beneficent image of penicillin. The widely publicized record of its effectiveness against serious infections had lent great credence to the popular notion that American medicine had achieved its "Golden Age." "Highbrow and mass media commentators alike," historian of medicine John C. Burnham has noted, "associated medical practice with the 'miracles' of science and made few adverse comments on the profession." "By the 1940's," he added, "virtually everyone had heard of miracle drugs and many people knew that they owed their lives to them." Despite criticisms of "political activities" of the American Medical Association, the public continued to praise the efforts of the medical profession. Although wartime Americans may have resented Chester Keefer's strict control of penicillin, public reverence for the fruits of modern medicine was perhaps never greater than during the postwar years.[27]

While the lay public looked to the marvels of penicillin, the federal government considered the postwar role of researchers who had served the nation during wartime. The war years had demonstrated that a close relationship between the federal government and the academic community could enhance national security. The clinical investigation of penicillin, just as the Manhattan Project, had shown the importance of a close alliance between the federal government and academia. Could this relationship produce similar results in peacetime as well? By the Kennedy years, Barry Karl noted, the federal government had acquired "a cadre of academic specialists" from every discipline who functioned both as advisors and directors of national policy. "Managerial elites" had become a crucial part of modern liberal democracy.[28]

During the final years of the war, the Roosevelt administration considered postwar funding for medical and scientific research. Even before the bombing of Hiroshima and Nagasaki, OSRD director Vannevar Bush released *Science, The Endless Frontier*, in which he addressed four issues: 1) Within the guidelines of military security, how should postwar America disseminate its scientific advances? 2) How could the government most effectively continue its support of research projects? 3) What role should the government play in supporting public and private research? 4) How might the nation develop a plan to encourage younger scientists to pursue research careers?[29]

The American research establishment was in an excellent position to continue wartime projects. Few could deny the numerous wartime medical and scientific advances. As one summer 1945 editorial announced, "Tanks, fire bombs, Superfortresses, fast fighter planes, radar, sulfa drugs, penicillin, blood plasma, and all other weapons which are helping the Allies win the war and keep down the death rate are the contributions of scientists." These medical and scientific advances seemed all the more exciting in light of the generally upbeat mood that accompanied the end of the Second World War. Science, Roosevelt had hoped, might provide national security and an improved standard of living for postwar Americans.[30]

While politicians and newspaper editors debated whether a postwar scientific agency should be placed under the wing of the federal government (as in the case of the OSRD, NDRC, and CMR), Bush's concern in *Science, The Endless Frontier* remained: government support of science was of inestimable value to postwar America and the postwar world. Bush argued that only the physical, biological, and medical sciences be included within the postwar research establishment. In his opinion, these disciplines had made the greatest contribution to wartime research. The social sciences, as policy makers had contended during the days of the Science Advisory Board of the 1930s, lacked the objectivity of the "hard" sciences—biology, physics, chemistry, etc. Hadn't medical researchers brought penicillin from the laboratory to the bedside? Hadn't physicists and engineers perfected the atomic bomb? Although social scientists had contributed to the war effort, Bush and his colleagues believed that their work could not match the record of the biological and physical sciences. Newspaper editorials also praised Bush's stand. One writer boasted that Bush's proposal was not a "scheme to control the manners, morals, and mores of the people. In short, 'social science' is not involved."[31]

The government-supported "hard" sciences, Bush added, could maintain international peace by giving the United States a strategic advantage against its enemies. The scientific community could focus its attention on medicine, detection devices, and weaponry that would provide a better life for all—in war or peace. Bush emphasized that his proposal enhanced national security, well-being, and overall "cultural progress."[32]

Production and clinical investigation of penicillin represented an invaluable facet of the wartime research program. By the end of the war, Department of Agriculture engineers and biochemists had perfected penicillin's large-scale manufacture, providing adequate supplies of the drug for military and civilian needs. The rapidity with which penicillin emerged from low-yield surface culture production to huge vats inspired one contemporary to dub penicillin "Science's Cinderella."[33]

The issue of governmentally funded research programs rekindled an important question that had plagued the COC: academic freedom. The wartime agenda had required that scientists focus upon areas of military concern, and many scientists (although there clearly were exceptions in the clinical investigation of penicillin) accepted these restrictions. Would these limitations remain in peacetime? Academic freedom, Bush believed, meant free inquiry. He added that "scientific progress" in the national interest required "the free play of free intellects, working on subjects of their own choice, in the manner dictated by their curiosity for the exploration of the unknown," a position that echoed the Science Advisory Board a decade earlier. One of his greatest fears had been (and remained) the control of scientific research by politicians rather than scientists. Politician-directed research, Bush reiterated, had no place in a democracy.[34]

A. N. Richards echoed this same sentiment in a 1946 *Science* article. He wrote, "To provide for the future advance of science and the true discoveries which will inevitably accrue, it is only necessary that the present generation of productive scientists be given freedom from intellectual restrictions, optimal facilities, and discriminatingly selected disciples." Kenneth M. Endicott and Ernest M. Allen added in 1953 that postwar U.S. Public Health Service (USPHS) grants strove to guard the autonomy of the researchers. They noted, "The investigator works on problems of his own choosing and is not obliged to adhere to a preconceived plan. He is free to publish as he chooses and to change his research without clearance if he finds new and more promising leads." "Once a grant is made," the authors concluded confidently, "there is no direction or interference on the part of the Government."[35]

Similarly, on the issue of medical research, John R. Steelman called for the federal government to continue its support of basic and applied research through medical schools. Federal assistance, he believed, encouraged biomedical research which could then be used for the betterment of the American people. Without a solid research base, Steelman stressed, America's standard of medical education would suffer enormously. He concluded, "The scientific world is of one mind that fundamental research in medicine must be continued and augmented, as in all other sciences. Only institutions with substantial resources can afford to support it comprehensively." (Indeed, the basic sciences had played an integral role in making the penicillin effort a success.) Steelman went even farther several years later when he called for support in excess of $300 million dollars annually. Without adequate funding, he wrote, the "precarious financial situation" of many medical schools threatened to curtail promising research programs. Chester Keefer reiterated this sentiment, noting that "more and more basic research is required if we are to conquer the existing diseases and the new diseases that are appearing, because, like human beings, new diseases are born, they thrive and die."[36]

Vannevar Bush also understood the importance of medical research and American medical schools for the postwar era. These institutions had, after all, supplied many of the researchers for wartime projects—not least the study of penicillin. Bush attributed this situation to university endowments and grants made in the years prior to the war. Inadequate postwar funding, however, was threatening the esteemed position of the United States within the international community, and—far worse—might slow medical progress to a crawl. To fill the gap, Bush requested substantial funding for basic research through grants (similar to those that the government had awarded during the war years) to medical schools and universities alike. During the early postwar years, the National Institutes of Health (NIH), the National Cancer Institute (NCI), various divisions of the United States Public Health Service (USPHS), and the newly created National Institute of Mental Health (NIMH) all flourished under a flood of government support.[37]

The penicillin effort influenced the course of postwar NIH research. Given the effectiveness of the antibiotics against acute bacterial illnesses, the NIH shifted its attention to chronic diseases. Surgeon General Thomas Parran in a 1947 speech before Congress observed that increased longevity had created "an aging population" in the United States. Since the antibiotics had lowered the mortality rates for many infectious diseases, the "relative importance of the chronic diseases and the disabling conditions of later life has increased correspondingly," he noted. Cancer and cardiovascular disease, Parran continued, had become the primary causes of death in the United States. The former, he predicted, "will increase with the increasing proportion of older people in our population unless more effective means are found to check it."[38]

The hopes of Vannevar Bush and other leaders of the American medical and scientific community bore fruit as the number of medical researchers expanded nearly 30 percent between 1944 and 1949. Of those, the majority held medical school posts. Far more striking, the total expenditure in support of medical research increased ten-fold between 1941 ($18 million) and 1951 ($181 million). The federal government, "a very minor contributor" at the beginning of the war, had increased its support of basic research from $28 million in 1946 to $76 million in 1951.[39]

Funding for medical research increased so that the pool of researchers had risen "more rapidly than the general population, and that expenditures for medical research have increased at a greater rate than national income." Between 1945 and 1950 the funding for the USPHS alone increased from over $85,000 to nearly $13 million. By 1953, that amount had reached over $20 million.[40]

Increased funding had lured more and more individuals into scientific careers. "Educational institutions and hospitals that never before participated in research," Kenneth Endicott and Ernest Allen commented in 1953, "are beginning to appoint research-minded staff members who attract research money, train young men, and so forth." Indeed, funding was producing positive results, and the authors noted increases in medical scientific publications between 1948 and 1951 of nearly 50 percent from government laboratories, nearly 30 percent from universities and colleges, and nearly 20 percent from research foundations.[41]

Increased postwar funding also had a positive effect on the geographic distribution of researchers. Between 1944 and 1949, for example, the number of medical scientists working in areas *other than* the New England and the Middle Atlantic states had increased at an unprecedented rate. Furthermore, federal funding also provided medical schools and universities that were far from the long-established Eastern institutions with a source of research support. Penicillin rationing through the OCPD and its depot hospitals may well have been one catalyst of this trend.[42]

The wartime work of the COC members, which brought them directly in contact with federally funded research, also resulted in a postwar effect as COC members assumed postwar policy making positions. Chester Keefer, for example, served the Eisenhower Administration as a special advisor to the secretary of the Department of Health, Education, and Welfare; he also oversaw the rationing of streptomycin in the late 1940s and the polio vaccine during the 1950s. Francis Blake and Barry Wood both served on the Armed Forces Epidemiological Board, E. K. Marshall became an advisor to the National Cancer Institute, and Perrin Long acted as a consultant to the Veterans Adminstration, the Food and Drug Administration, and the USPHS. Donald Anderson also held a variety of posts, including consultant to the army surgeon general from 1953 to 1966, and served on the President's Science Advisory Committee on Bioastronautics from 1961 to 1966.[43]

The wartime experiences of COC members also advanced their reputations. Francis Blake, for example, continued to guide the Department of Medicine at Yale until his death in early 1952. Perrin Long, the first chairman of the COC, remained at Johns Hopkins before moving to the State University of New York's Downstate Medical Center in Brooklyn in 1951. Barry Wood remained at Washington University before moving to Johns Hopkins in 1955; John Lockwood accepted a professorship in 1946 at the Columbia University College of Physicians and Surgeons; and Champ Lyons went to Tulane University in 1945 where he was appointed associate professor of surgery. Chester Keefer accepted a position as Dean of Boston University Medical School in 1955.[44]

Donald Anderson, although not formally a member of the COC, also benefited from his role in the wartime penicillin program. As a medical resident, he had gained administrative experience in handling penicillin requests in Keefer's absence and had published nearly a dozen papers on the drug's use by the end of the war. In 1945, Anderson accepted a position as dean and assistant professor of medicine at Boston University. By the early 1950s, he had taken a post as Dean and Professor of Medicine at the University of Rochester School of Medicine and Dentistry. He co-authored *The Therapeutic Value of Penicillin: A Study of 10,000 Cases* with Chester Keefer in 1948.[45]

The wartime penicillin program also influenced the growth of the postwar antibiotic industry. Both the domestic and international sales of postwar penicillin had expanded rapidly during the mid-1940s. Although the United States had exported only 29 billion units in 1944, the quota rose to 721.6 billion units by late summer 1945. "Penicillin, thus," Robert Coghill and Roy Koch commented in 1945, "has helped to establish a better understanding among nations, which should aid in the establishment of world peace." The United States even considered sharing penicillin fermentation technology with the Soviet Union as a gesture of postwar good will and cooperation—a plan that folded with rising Cold War tensions.[46]

Streptomycin, chloramphenicol, and Aureomycin had joined penicillin by the early 1950s. These new antibiotics had provided effective treatment for diseases against which even penicillin had no effect. "Equal to [penicillin's] importance as a drug has been the effect of precipitating and sustaining the unprecedented search for other drugs of microbial origin," Kenneth Raper commented in 1952. Since penicillin had been extracted from the common *Penicillium* mold, researchers considered the possibility of discovering similar substances. "Everywhere the searchers say:" Kenneth Raper added, " 'If it can happen once, surely it can happen again'." In the same way that *Penicillium* mold had proven destructive to a broad range of microorganisms, actinomycetes, a common soil fungus, spawned "the next four clinically outstanding antibiotics," streptomycin, chloramphenicol, Aureomycin, and Terramycin. Each of the drugs complemented the action of penicillin and, in some cases, actually surpassed it.[47]

Streptomycin followed penicillin at the close of the war. Early clinical trials proved that it effectively treated penicillin-resistant gram-negative organisms and also "was found to have a suppressive effect upon the growth of the tubercle bacillus in man." The wartime experiences of drug manufacturers had provided them with invaluable experience in large-scale antibiotic production, which they deftly applied to the study and manufacture of streptomycin. Drawing upon wartime experience with submerged culture technology, drug companies initiated mass production by the late 1940s.[48]

Streptomycin, however, remained extremely scarce during the early postwar years. As a result, the COC accepted responsibility for its investigation and rationed the drug in much the same fashion as wartime penicillin. The COC's wartime experience, combined with the importance of following research protocol, required that physicians use streptomycin only according to specific clinical criteria. In May 1946, the *Journal of the American Medical Association* published the COC's "Official Statement Concerning Streptomycin." These guidelines, authored by Chester Keefer, outlined the goals of the COC's streptomycin trials: to determine the proper clinical use of the drug and investigate its potential toxicity. He stressed that "much remains to be learned concerning limitations of the usefulness, methods of administration, dosage, toxicity, and so on." In order to acquire as much information as possible, Keefer concluded, the COC would need to restrict most of the drug to its team of accredited investigators, many of whom had participated in wartime penicillin research.[49]

Small amounts of streptomycin would go to individual physicians who had patients under their care who might benefit from the new drug. Keefer emphasized, however, that his Committee required complete "bacteriological diagnosis of the case. . . . and when streptomycin is allotted it is with the understanding that a full report of the case is to be returned to the committee for analysis and that all unused material is to be returned for use in other suitable cases."[50]

Keefer, just as he had during the penicillin investigations, stressed the importance of the proper use of streptomycin and requested that unused portions of the drug be returned promptly for distribution to other patients. All too often millions of units of penicillin had disappeared mysteriously or been given to patients whose illnesses were not penicillin-sensitive. Keefer reiterated that the limited supply of streptomycin made it "obvious that patients selected to receive it must be those whom it can be expected to benefit and from whose treatment useful, needed information can be derived." The "sole purpose" of the COC's program lay in "obtaining the necessary information concerning streptomycin in the shortest possible time."[51]

Keefer emphasized that the COC had a particular "responsibility . . . to direct the investigation toward those infections that were most likely to be benefitted by it and to those that were resistant to penicillin and the sulfonamides." Commenting on a list of diseases that the Committee believed were streptomycin-sensitive, the COC chairman concluded, "It is the hope of the Committee that adequate ways and means may be found for studying the application of streptomycin to tuberculosis so that its place in the treatment of this disease can be defined."[52]

By the fall of 1946 the COC and its investigators had made significant progress toward determining the clinical indications of streptomycin. Studies had shown that the drug was useful in cases of tularemia, *Hemophilus influenzae* infection, and gram-negative infections of the urinary tract, bacteremia, and meningitis. Investigators also achieved promising results in pulmonary infections resulting from Friedlander's bacillus and other gram-negative microbes. Between March 1 and September 1, 1946, the COC allocated fifty-five kilograms of streptomycin to accredited investigators and private practitioners. By November 30 of that year the Committee had received case reports on over 2,800 patients.[53]

Keefer once again faced an onslaught of desperate individuals who tried to obtain streptomycin for themselves, their family members, or their friends. It is likely that the popular press, which ran sensational reports of the new "wonder drug," fueled the flood of these petitions. Keefer denied these requests, many of which were from persons suffering from tuberculosis, because they were for diseases that were not under investigation at that time. "The original policy as agreed upon at the beginning of the program in March [1, 1946] concerning tuberculosis was maintained throughout the period and no exceptions were made," Keefer stressed. Although existing evidence had suggested the usefulness of streptomycin against tuberculosis, the COC elected to postpone study of this disease until clinicians could locate a suitable population for long-range study. Keefer noted that the proper investigation of tuberculosis "would require a large number of patients who could be followed most carefully for a period of several years."[54]

The COC realized early on that tuberculosis represented "one of the most important problems" facing the clinical investigation of streptomycin. Only TB patients that had received streptomycin prior to March 1, 1946 were given additional amounts of the drug. The new drug had created quite an excitement in the lay and professional community alike. Keefer noted that the COC's paper, "Streptomycin in the Treatment of Infections: A Report of One Thousand Cases" had attracted "several hundred requests" for reprints from physicians "all over the country and additional requests arrive daily." He concluded, "The mail continues to pour in consisting of requests for streptomycin . . . for patients unable to afford it, requests for the treatment of tuberculosis, requests from hospitals who wish to be designated as depots, as well as numerous inquiries for advice concerning the handling of individual patients."[55]

Streptomycin had its limits. The drug had little effect on typhoid, brucellosis, and salmonella. Streptomycin, just as penicillin, had also caused allergic reactions ranging from urticaria to headache and fever in some patients. Clinical investigators noted also that *Staphylococcus aureus* superinfections often occurred during streptomycin treatment.[56]

The evolution of the streptomycin rationing policy followed a course similar to that of wartime penicillin rationing. However, centralized control—which greatly facilitated distribution—did not have the same effect in the postwar era. At first, centralized control of the new drug proved feasible, since so little of the substance was available. A single coordinator dispensed the drug to selected clinicians who then selected cases among Veterans Administration hospital patients. The small number of researchers operating within a centralized system worked well—despite objections by the image-conscious VA that clinicians were "experimenting" on veterans.[57]

This system, however, deteriorated as the supply of streptomycin increased, and the popular press touted the wonders of the new drug. As a result, patients, physicians, and hospitals throughout the United States clamored for streptomycin. Without the war as justification, many asked, how could the COC deny anyone the drug? Extending investigations to a wider sphere of hospitals, however, might have compromised the early stages of the clinical research program.[58]

Policy makers reasoned that regional administration, similar to the Office of Civilian Penicillin Distribution's rationing system, provided a viable alternative as supplies of the drug had increased to a point where centralized control of streptomycin was no longer feasible, but *decentralized* distribution might result in its improper use. One contemporary observer feared that politicians might "attempt to break down the investigative program into one of purely therapy." Clinical investigation—not "therapy"—Keefer had stressed during the penicillin trials, remained the primary purpose of the research program. As increasing numbers of VA hospitals became involved in the streptomycin studies, safeguarding of clinical protocol grew increasingly difficult. Harry Marks noted, "Once decisions about eligibility were decentralized, moral suasion provided the principal means for ensuring that participating investigators were following the research protocol." By 1947, the streptomycin investigations had returned to the tried-and-true cooperative clinical protocol.[59]

The war effort had made the selection of patients a relatively simple matter for the COC. Patients were chosen according to their clinical diagnosis. Although many patients objected when the

Committee denied them penicillin, the wartime emergency helped to justify case selection. The clinicians who investigated streptomycin, however, lacked such justification. They could argue only that their research was in the interest of the advancement of science. To select patients, clinicians divided them into cases that received treatment and those that did not. If the condition of a patient in the untreated group deteriorated, investigators could petition an Appeals Board which then decided whether or not the patient would receive streptomycin.[60]

Streptomycin trials differed from the penicillin research in another way. Patients in the nontreatment group were not informed that their physician had knowingly withheld a life-saving drug. Without the wartime emergency to justify denying streptomycin for some patients, the issue smacked of experimentation—without the knowledge of the patient. Could an investigator, in the interest of clinical protocol, deny a patient a drug that might well save his life? Apparently so. Harry Marks commented that this ethic of cooperative clinical research and the random selection of cases (notable in later streptomycin studies) became commonplace in postwar clinical investigations.[61]

By 1950, other antibiotics had joined penicillin and streptomycin. Chloramphenicol, isolated from soil organisms found in Venezuela, appeared in 1947. Effective in the treatment of typhoid fever, it also proved useful against typhus and Rocky Mountain Spotted Fever. Aureomycin, complementing the antimicrobial spectra of penicillin, streptomycin, and chloramphenicol, followed in the summer of 1948. One contemporary study suggested that the drug represented "the most important antibiotic developed since the introduction of penicillin." Terramycin, introduced in early 1950, also represented an important addition to the antibiotic pharmacopoeia. It effectively treated penicillin-resistant syphilis and produced "favorable responses" in cases of amebiasis and brucellosis. By the 1960s, a number of semisynthetic penicillins, such as ampicillin, had also been developed.[62]

The introduction of additional postpenicillin antibiotics continued to raise concerns about the overuse of these drugs. Few doctors seemed willing to take the time to type the infecting organism and then determine the drug best able to treat the condition. The proliferation of the new antibiotics by the early 1950s forced infectious disease experts to reemphasize the careful use of these drugs. Echoing the wartime clinical guidelines of the COC, one concerned physician recommended that all medical students and residents "should receive systematic education in the field of antibiotics." Only a comprehensive knowledge of the clinical indications of these drugs, one clinician wrote in the mid-1950s, permitted physicians to determine "*when, what,* and *how* to prescribe antibiotic therapy." He also emphasized a final point, for he understood the role of patients in the overprescription of antibiotics: "Proper ways and means should be found to educate the lay-public to abandon . . . the common practice of demanding antibiotic medication from their physician."[63]

Other studies presented similar evidence of the growth of "antibiotic abandon." The *Journal of the American Medical Association*, for example, reported in 1953 that many physicians commonly prescribed antibiotics for patients suffering from viral respiratory infections such as the common cold. It was clear, the study concluded, that none of the antibiotics had any effect on such cases. Another investigator warned that physicians might soon be faced with infections resistant to all known antibiotics. Furthermore, surviving family members had filed lawsuits by the late 1950s for "fatal reaction to penicillin." Even chloramphenicol, one of the most promising of the new antibiotics, had been linked to depressed bone marrow function and aplastic anemia. These episodes, James Whorton commented, "forcefully reaffirmed one of medicine's perpetual truths, that there are no safe drugs, only safe physicians."[64]

The grave admonitions throughout the 1950s and 1960s, however, had little immediate effect on the improper prescription of antibiotics. One 1974 study noted that older physicians, many of whom had entered the medical profession in the 1940s and 1950s continued to prescribe these drugs more freely than their younger colleagues. These younger doctors had begun to return to the clinical prudence stressed by Keefer and the COC several decades earlier. Another survey from the mid-1970s found that over 90 percent of residents believed that private practitioners overprescribed antibiotics. Of this group, nearly two-thirds added that these physicians "significantly" overused them. While this does not suggest that they would not overuse antibiotics, it does indicate a greater awareness of the problem of overprescription.[65]

Nor did the wartime example of the COC influence the immediate postwar use of antibiotics. Practicing physicians, weary of the wartime restrictions on penicillin, embarked upon a "spree" of "antibiotic abandon." Aware of the "miracle cures" that resulted from treatment with antibiotics, laypersons pressured their physician for one of these drugs. Practitioners and patients alike seemed to show relatively little concern over resistant bacterial strains and dangerous allergic reactions.

By the 1970s rationing of medical resources had attracted increasing attention. Although some medical professionals argued that "rationing" represented "an odious concept, and life would be better if social planners found some other occupation with which to concern themselves," it became difficult to escape allocative decisions. The primary question, therefore, became not one of whether medical resources should be distributed but how this should be done in the interest of "dignified care," "equity," and "efficiency."[66]

The problems that surrounded the rationing of the early antibiotics have reappeared most recently in the clinical trials of AZT. During the initial use of this drug, familiar issues arose. First, use of the drug was restricted to physicians known for their experience in treating AIDS patients. Among their cases, only those that met specific criteria would receive AZT. Burroughs Wellcome, the company that manufactures AZT, emphasized several goals in 1987: to acquire as much clinical data as quickly as possible, to distribute the drug only to patients who might benefit from it, and to prevent blackmarket availability of AZT.[67]

The wartime penicillin effort also demonstrated the ways in which researchers, well funded by government, could serve national policy needs. The members of the COC represented only a fraction of the many Ph.D.'s and M.D.'s who accepted positions as advisors of American scientific and medical research policy. The example of wartime penicillin, however, confirmed the important roles which academics could play in both war and peace.

Finally, the development of penicillin spurred interest in other antimicrobial drugs. Scarcely a decade after the war's end American pharmaceutical companies had placed a number of additional antibiotics on the market. Although penicillin remains a useful drug, antibiotics such as Terramycin, Aureomycin, and chloramphenicol have their usefulness against infections that are penicillin-resistant. Few of these drugs have had the powerful effect on the public mind as "the wonder drug of 1943," penicillin.

Notes

1. James C. Whorton, " 'Antibiotic Abandon': The Resurgence of Therapeutic Rationalism," in John Parascandola, ed., *The History of Antibiotics: A Symposium* (Madison, Wis., 1979), 125-136.

2. See especially Daniel S. Greenberg, *The Politics of Pure Science* (New York, 1967); Margaret Rossiter, "Science and Public Policy since World War II," *Osiris* 2d series, 1 (1985): 273-294.

3. Gina Kolata, "Imminent Marketing of AZT Raises Problems," *Science* 235 (20 March 1987): 1462-1463; Chester S. Keefer, "Official Statement Concerning Streptomycin," *Journal of the American Medical Association* 131 (4 May 1946): 31.

4. Harry F. Dowling, *Fighting Infection: Conquests of the Twentieth Century*, (Cambridge, Mass., 1977), 142; Wesley W. Spink, *Infectious Diseases: Prevention and Treatment in the Nineteenth and Twentieth Centuries*, 283; H. R. S. Harley, J. A. Baty, and J. H. Bowie, "The Pathogenicity of Penicillin-Insensitive Infection," *British Medical Journal* 1 (27 April 1946): 639, 643; Robert S. Fielding and Frank B. Queen, "Strain Variations in Penicillin Sensitivity Among Bacterial Species Encountered in War Wounds and Infections," *American Journal of Clinical Pathology* 16 (1946): 63.

5. Donald G. Anderson and Chester S. Keefer, *The Therapeutic Value of Penicillin: A Study of 10,000 Cases* (Ann Arbor, Mich., 1948), 128.

6. Harry J. Robinson, "Toxicity and Efficacy of Penicillin," *Journal of Pharmacology and Experimental Therapeutics* 77 (January 1943): 70-79; Dorothy M. Hamre, et al., "The Toxicity of Penicillin as Prepared for Clinical Use," *American Journal of Medical Science* 206 (November 1943): 642-652; Chester S. Keefer to A. N. Richards, 29 April 1943, Committee on Medical Research Files, Record Group 227, National Archives, Washington, D.C. [hereafter cited as CMR, RG 227].

7. Chester S. Keefer to A. N. Richards, 29 April 1943; Champ Lyons to A.N. Richards, 2 August 1943; "Memorandum on Penicillin," 31 August 1943, CMR, RG 227.

8. A. Neish Barker, "Allergic Reactions to Penicillin," *The Lancet* 1 (10 February 1945): 178; Anderson and Keefer, *The Therapeutic Value of Penicillin*, 127.

9. Adolph Rostenberg, Jr., and Henry Welch, "A Study of the Types of Hypersensitivity Induced by Penicillin," *American Journal of Medical Science* 210 (August 1945): 167; Chester S. Keefer, "Penicillin—Its Present Status in the Treatment of Infections," *American Journal of Medical Science* 210 (August 1945): 155.

10. "Certification of Penicillin and Derivative Drugs," *Legislative History of the Federal Food, Drug, and Cosmetic Act and Its Amendments*, vol. 7, U.S. Department of Health, Education, and Welfare, 443; "Certification of Penicillin," *Legislative History*, 512. The FDA also oversaw the certification of streptomycin. See "Pretesting and Certification of Streptomycin," *Legislative History*, 512.

11. Anderson and Keefer, *The Therapeutic Value of Penicillin*, 284-288; Chester S. Keefer, "Penicillin: A Wartime Accomplishment," in E. C. Andrus et al., eds., *Advances in Military Medicine Made by American Investigators Working Under the Sponsorship of the Committee on Medical Research*, vol. II (Boston, 1948), 722.

12. Ethan Allan Brown, "Reactions to Penicillin: A Review of the Literature, 1943-1948," *Annals of Allergy* 6 (November-December 1948): 723-746; Lawrence Weld Smith and Ann Dolan Walker, *Penicillin Decade, 1941-1951: Sensitizations and Toxicities* (Washington, D.C., 1951).

13. Whorton, " 'Antibiotic Abandon,' " in Parascandola, ed., *The History of Antibiotics*, 131; Leslie A. Falk, "Will Penicillin Be Used Indiscriminately?" *New England Journal of Medicine* 127 (17 March 1945): 672; Leslie A. Falk, "Is the Indiscriminate Use of Penicillin Imminent?" *Journal of the American Pharmaceutical Association* 34 (1945): 126-127.

14. Whorton, " 'Antibiotic Abandon,' " in Parascandola, ed., *The History of Antibiotics*, 131.

15. *Ibid.*; Dowling, *Fighting Infection*, 241-242; Whorton, " 'Antibiotic Abandon,' " 129, 131 in Parascandola, ed., *The History of Antibiotics*; "Penicillin: Unexcelled and Now Obtainable," *New England Journal of Medicine* 232 (27 December 1945): 411; Peter Temin, *Taking Your Medicine: Drug Regulation in the United States* (Cambridge, Mass., 1980), 113-116; David P. Adams, "The Penicillin Mystique and the Popular Press (1935-1950)," *Pharmacy in History* 26 (1984): 134-142.

The Legacy of Wartime Penicillin Rationing

16. Temin, *Taking Your Medicine*, 115.

17. *Ibid.*, 115-116.

18. Richard H. Shryock, *American Medical Research: Past and Present* (New York, 1947); Dowling, *Fighting Infection*, 241; Jerry Avorn, Milton Chen, and Robert Hartley, "Scientific versus Commercial Sources of Influence on the Prescribing Behavior of Physicians," *American Journal of Medicine* 73 (July 1982): 4-8.

19. Quoted in Whorton, " 'Antibiotic Abandon,' " in Parascandola, ed. *The History of Antibiotics*, 129.

20. The Elixir Sulfanilamide tragedy of the late 1930s had already cast the sulfas in a negative light before the public eye. See Adams, "The Penicillin Mystique and the Popular Press (1935-1950)," 135-137; Boris Sokoloff, *The Miracle Drugs* (Chicago, 1949); Paul De Kruif, "Conquest of a Killer," *Reader's Digest*, March 1945, 27-31.

21. J. D. Ratcliff, *Yellow Magic: The Story of Penicillin* (New York, 1945), 163.

22. *Ibid.*, 160-167; "Cure by Toothpaste," *Newsweek*, 25 December 1945, 73.

23. "Penicillin in Lozenges," *Science News Letter*, 6 January 1945, 2.

24. Eric F. Goldman, *The Crucial Decade and After: 1945-1960* (New York, 1960), 11-14; Graham Greene, *The Third Man and the Fallen Idol* (London, 1964), 95-97; Lawrence P. Garrod, letter to the editor, *British Medical Journal* (28 September 1974): 805.

25. Quoted in Adams, "The Penicillin Mystique and the Popular Press," 140.

26. Quoted in *Ibid.*

27. John C. Burnham, "American Medicine's Golden Age: What Happened to It?," *Science* 215 (19 March 1982): 1474-1475.

28. Barry D. Karl, "Philanthropy, Policy Planning, and the Bureaucratization of the Democratic Ideal," *Daedalus* (1976): 129, 143; Stephen P. Strickland, *Politics, Science, and Dread Disease: A Short History of United States Medical Research* (Cambridge, Mass., 1972), 32-54; Daniel M. Fox, *Health Policies, Health Politics: The British and American Experience, 1911-1965* (Princeton, 1986), 149-168, 188-206; Kenneth MacDonald Jones, "The Endless Frontier," *Prologue* 8 (Spring 1976): 35-46; Vannevar Bush, *Science, the Endless Frontier* (Washington, D.C., 1945).

29. Jones, "The Endless Frontier," 36.

30. Quoted in *Ibid.*, 37.

31. *Ibid.*, 42. For a discussion of the Science Advisory Board, see Lewis Auerbach, "Scientists in the New Deal: A Pre-War Episode in the Relations Between Science and Government in the United States," *Minerva* (1965): 457-482.

32. Quoted in Jones, "The Endless Frontier," 42.

33. Robert D. Coghill, "Penicillin: Science's Cinderella," *Chemical and Engineering News* 22 (25 April 1944): 593.

34. Bush, *Science, the Endless Frontier*, 7; Lewis Auerbach, "Scientists in the New Deal," 457-482; Robert Kargon and Elizabeth Hodes, "Karl Compton, Isaiah Bowman, and the Politics of Science in the Great Depression," *Isis* 76 (September 1985): 301-318.

35. A. N. Richards, "The Impact of the War on Medicine," *Science* 103 (10 May 1946): 578; Kenneth M. Endicott and Ernest M. Allen, "The Growth of Medical Research 1941-1953 and the Role of Public Health Service Research Grants," *Science* 118 (25 September 1953): 341.

36. James L. Penick, Jr., et al., eds., *The Politics of American Science, 1939 to the Present* (Chicago, 1965), 112-116; Chester S. Keefer, *Medical Science and Society* (Boston, 1956), 14.

37. *Ibid.*, 114, 119; Strickland, *Politics, Science and Dread Disease*.

38. Quoted in Penick et al., eds., *The Politics of American Science*, 122-123; Victoria A. Harden, *Inventing the NIH: Federal Biomedical Research Policy, 1887-1937* (Baltimore, 1986), 183. For a recent discussion of the image of cancer in American society, see James T. Patterson, *The Dread Disease: Cancer and Modern American Culture* (Cambridge, Mass., 1987).

39. Endicott and Allen, "The Growth of Medical Research," 337.

40. *Ibid.*

41. *Ibid.*, 338.

42. *Ibid.*, 339.

43. "Dr. Keefer Named to Health Post by Eisenhower," *Boston Globe*, [summer 1953?]; "Dr. Chester S. Keefer, 74, Ex-BU Dean, Hospital Chief," *Boston Herald*, 4 February 1972, clippings in Boston University Medical Library Archives, Boston, Mass.; "The Doctors Arrive," *Newsweek*, 17 August 1953, 58; Keefer, *Medical Science and Society*; John Rodman Paul, "Francis Gilman Blake, 1887-1952," (1954): 16-17; "Wood, William Barry, Jr.," in Martin Kaufman, Stuart Galishoff, and Todd L. Savitt, eds., *Dictionary of American Medical Biography*, vol. II (Westport, CT., 1984), 822-823; Thomas H. Maren, "Eli Kennerly Marshall, Jr., 1889-1966," *Bulletin of the Johns Hopkins Hospital* 119 (October 1966): 251; Personal interview with Donald G. Anderson, Magnolia Springs, AL, 5 January 1985.

44. Paul, "Francis Gilman Blake," 14-18; "Wood, William Barry, Jr.," 822-823; "A Verray Parfit Praktisour," *Medical Times* 94 (June 1966): 696-698; "Lockwood, John S(alem)," in Jacques Cattell, ed., *American Men of Science* (Lancaster, Penn., 1949), 1515; "Lyons, Dr. Champ," in Jacques Cattell, ed., *American Men of Science*, 1552.

45. Personal interview with Donald G. Anderson, 5 January 1985.

46. Robert D. Coghill and Roy S. Koch, "Penicillin—A Wartime Accomplishment," *Chemical and Engineering News* 23 (1946): 2310-2316; Patricia Spain Ward, "Antibiotics and International Relations after World War II," in Parascandola, ed., *The History of Antibiotics*, 101-112; Hobby, *Penicillin: Meeting the Challenge*, 250.

47. Kenneth B. Raper, "A Decade of Antibiotics in America," *Mycologia* 44 (January-February 1952): 15-16.

48. *Ibid.*, 15-21.

49. Keefer, "Official Statement Concerning Streptomycin," 31; see also Harry M. Marks, "Notes from the Underground: The Social Organization of Therapeutic Research," in Russell C. Maulitz and Diana E. Long, eds., *Grand Rounds: One Hundred Years of Internal Medicine* (Philadelphia, 1988), esp. 312-320.

50. Keefer, "Official Statement Concerning Streptomycin," 31.

51. *Ibid.*

52. Chester S. Keefer et al., "Streptomycin in the Treatment of Infections," *Journal of the American Medical Association* 132 (7 September 1946): 4-5.

53. *Ibid.*; "Clinical Investigation of Streptomycin by the Committee on Chemotherapy of the National Research Council," 30 November 1946, 1, 3,

Committees on Military Medicine Files, Committee on Chemotherapeutic and Other Agents, National Academy of Sciences, Washington, D.C. [hereafter cited as COMM, NAS].

54. *Ibid.*, 1-2.

55. *Ibid.*, 2-3.

56. Chester S. Keefer et al., "Streptomycin in the Treatment of Infections," *Journal of the American Medical Association* 132 (14 September 1946): 74-77.

57. Marks, "Notes from the Underground," in Maulitz and Long, eds., *Grand Rounds*, 313.

58. *Ibid.*

59. *Ibid.*, 313-320.

60. *Ibid.*

61. *Ibid.*

62. Hobby, *Penicillin: Meeting the Challenge*, 230-231.

63. Whorton, " 'Antibiotic Abandon,' " in Parascandola, ed., *The History of Antibiotics*, 129-130; Allen E. Hussar, "A Proposed Crusade for the Rational Use of Antibiotics," *Antibiotics Annual* (1954-1955): 381-382.

64. Philip N. Jones, Roy S. Bigham, and Phil R. Manning, "Use of Antibiotics in Nonbacterial Respiratory Infections," *Journal of the American Medical Association* 153 (26 September 1953): 264; Harry F. Dowling, "The Effect of the Emergence of Resistant Strains on the Future of Antibiotic Therapy," *Antibiotics Annual* (1953-1954): 33; Perrin H. Long, "Fatal Anaphylactic Reactions to Penicillin," *Antibiotics Annual* (1953-1954): 35-40; Abraham Rosenthal, "Follow-Up Study of Fatal Penicillin Reactions," *Journal of the American Medical Association* 167 (28 June 1958): 1120; Whorton, " 'Antibiotic Abandon,' " in Parascandola, ed., *The History of Antibiotics*, 131-134.

65. 'Nea D'Amelio, "Are Family Doctors Prescribing Too Many Antibiotics?" *Medical Times* 102 (January 1974): 53-61; Nea D'Amelio, "What Young Doctors Told Us About Antibiotic Overkill," *Medical Times* (March 1974): 146; see also Henry E. Simmons and Paul D. Stolley, "This Is Medical Progress? Trends and Consequences of Antibiotic Use in the United States," *Journal of the American Medical Association* 227 (4 March 1974): 1023-1028.

66. David Mechanic, "The Growth of Medical Technology and Bureaucracy: Implications for Medical Care," 55 *Milbank Memorial Fund Quarterly* (Winter 1977): 61-78; David Mechanic, "Rationing Health Care: Public Policy and the Medical Marketplace," *Hastings Center Report* (February 1976): 34-37; David Mechanic, "How Should Medical Care Be Rationed?" *American Journal of Medicine* 68 (January 1979): 8-9.

67. Kolata, "Imminent Marketing of AZT Raises Problems," 1462-1463.

Conclusion

Wartime penicillin rationing held important lessons for American society. Foremost, the policies of the COC and the OCPD tested the ability of bureaucratic techniques to distribute scarce medical resources. By the late 1940s, the COC had demonstrated that objective clinical guidelines could successfully undergird an effective, efficient, and equitable rationing system. Moreover, the Committee had succeeded in collecting invaluable data on the clinical use of penicillin and streptomycin. Despite some lay and professional objections, the COC had selected a distribution system ideally suited to contemporary ideas about clinical investigation and the role of the State.

The guidelines of the COC allowed wartime physicians to detach themselves from the poignant situation of many of their patients. In the face of the COC's "policy," physicians could absolve themselves of any personal culpability resulting from their treating one case but not another. Any "blame" lay with the bureaucratic authority structure itself, not with the doctor. Masked by a shroud of professionalism, physicians could salve their consciences with the belief that their decisions reflected objective clinical criteria rather than personal judgment.[1]

Some wartime clinicians were unwilling to comply completely with treatment criteria. Haunted by the death of his son from bacterial endocarditis, Ward MacNeal continued to treat this disease with penicillin—even though Chester Keefer refused to authorize the drug for it. Martin Henry Dawson and Leo Loewe also dosed bacterial endocarditis cases with the drug. Although the "humanitarian" motives of MacNeal, Dawson, and Loewe were admirable, their disregard for COC policy undermined the impartial rationing of the drug. Keefer feared that news of their actions might bring allegations that he did not equitably allocate penicillin.

Moreover, any deviation from the investigative program of the COC (such as in the treatment of SBE or Wallace Herrell's desire to follow his own research agenda) also jeopardized the ethic of cooperative clinical investigation that tried to insure reliable, unbiased data.[2]

The treatment of bacterial endocarditis cases diverted large amounts of penicillin from cases known at that time to be penicillin-sensitive. Had L. W. Gorham not misused the drug, enough penicillin might have been available to save the two young children that died under John Lockwood's care in the summer of 1943. Only in the unusual case of Duncan Hallock did Chester Keefer violate his own treatment guidelines. One wonders if Eleanor Roosevelt's interest in the case (combined with the growing supply of penicillin by late 1943) mollified Keefer's typically rigid adherence to the COC's program. His curt letter to the First Lady concerning the Hallock case made it appear that the Committee chairman believed the drug would have no effect on ulcerative colitis.[3]

Although the COC equitably rationed penicillin, the OCPD allowed subjective considerations to color its distribution of the drug. Despite the efforts of the Task Committee on Civilian Distribution to maintain the COC's equitable distribution program, policymakers denied institutionalized mentally retarded, alcoholic, aged, and tubercular patients ready access to penicillin. Physicians who treated these individuals could obtain penicillin from a nearby depot hospital, however the OCPD had neglected to allocate the drug specifically for their use. Furthermore, the cost of penicillin, combined with the price of hospitalization, undoubtedly created hardships for poor patients.[4]

The purpose of this study has not been an analysis of the ethical principles that guided penicillin rationing, however the evidence clearly suggests that the COC distributed the drug according to utilitarian considerations. As the distribution criteria of the COC indicate, only those patients who stood to benefit from therapy—and whose treatment would provide useful data for the war effort—received the drug. In short, the Committee sought to provide the greatest good for the greatest number of individuals. Was the disease responsive to penicillin therapy? Would a sulfonamide provide a suitable alternative? If penicillin provided the only appropriate course of treatment, was the illness of military interest? Also, what was the prognosis of the patient? It made little sense, the COC reasoned, to treat patients who were moribund, thereby reducing the amount of the drug available for more promising cases.[5]

Subjective criteria had little bearing on the COC's rationing decisions. Only when the OCPD excluded institutionalized persons from convenient access to penicillin did inequity begin to cloud formulation or implementation of the drug's rationing. Penicillin requests seldom included information concerning race, marital status, or age. Although gender and area of residence often appeared on the petitions, the available data suggests that these criteria did not affect decisions to use (or not use) penicillin. In light of James Jones's study of the Tuskegee Syphilis Experiment, however, one wonders how many black Americans went untreated because their physicians did not even attempt to obtain penicillin.[6]

A pressing question remains: Did any viable alternatives exist to the COC's rationing policy? Might the Committee have selected cases at random, for example? Randomized case selection from a pool of potentially eligible patients would have lightened the emotional load on physicians who were responsible for penicillin rationing. It would have also lightened the intense pressure that weighed upon Keefer and the COC, thereby enabling clinical investigations to proceed even more smoothly. By randomly selecting patients, no single person or persons could be singled out as having direct control over distribution. A lottery would have helped to diminish the grim image of "Judge" Keefer.[7]

Randomization might also have provided more equitable access to penicillin. Only after the COC permitted private practitioners to use penicillin in late 1943 did the drug finally become, in theory at least, available to a wider array of patients. Prior to that time, only "accredited investigators" were able to use the drug, and the majority of them were affiliated with prestigious eastern medical schools. As of September 1943, nearly 60 percent of accredited investigators were located in the East. Moreover, they treated patients hospitalized in university medical centers.[8]

Random selection of cases might also have eased the emotional burden of the private practitioners who used penicillin. Keefer and his cadre of academics were accustomed to the rigors of clinical investigation, but many practicing physicians lacked such experience. Their task, as a result, would probably have been all the more difficult. Faced with a critically ill patient, many physicians must have asked, Why not at least *try* penicillin? They may have believed that they had a responsibility to do whatever was necessary to save the patient—regardless of the effect that treatment might have had on clinical guidelines.[9]

Private practitioners also regularly faced patients who begged for penicillin. Keefer's clinical setting insulated him more effectively from those who petitioned for penicillin; most of his petitioners were faceless persons who contacted him by telephone, telegram, or letter. The COC chairman, as a result, could keep himself protected from any personal contact with these patients. The practitioner, on the other hand, dealt directly with the family and friends of the gravely ill. Had the selection of cases been randomized, the attending physician's task might have been much easier. The decision to treat one patient over another would have rested not with the family doctor but with the lottery system. The necessity of denying treatment to one patient or another— especially when that decision was the result of another physician's waste of the scarce drug—must have touched even the most sober investigator.[10]

Random case selection, however, meshed poorly with contemporary assumptions about the function of the State. The rational, bureaucratic selection of eligible cases fit far more closely with administrative and intellectual trends of the FDR years. Bureaucracy provided an efficient means by which cases could be selected and treated and their clinical histories applied to future patients. This system also fit cooperative clinical research by allowing investigators to base treatment decisions solely on predetermined objective criteria and minimize ambiguity in case selection. Either a patient did—or did not—meet the necessary clinical criteria. Finally, the COC rationing system met with the approval of the legal counsel of the Office of Scientific Research and Development.[11]

One could argue that the bureaucratic rationing system utilized by the COC did not always grant equal consideration for treatment. Any inequities, however, lay in the necessity of support for the war effort. For example, researchers assigned—triaged, so to speak—some patients who might benefit from penicillin (such as those with osteomyelitis) to a waiting list where they remained indefinitely while the disease's degenerative process continued. For more acute infections, however, time often was of the essence. Since osteomyelitis typically was not life-threatening (and there were plenty of military cases for study), designating patients as "deserving" meant they would receive treatment as soon as ample supplies of penicillin became available. In the case of SBE, on the other hand, the deadly malady was not of military interest, nor did Keefer believe that penicillin could alter the course of the disease. Only after the drug's supplies increased—and certain renegade investigators used penicillin on SBE without Keefer's approval—did endocarditis cases receive treatment.

No matter how the COC or OCPD chose to ration penicillin, the public expressed shock at the life and death decisions that Keefer made. Health care remained in the public mind a market commodity to be bought and sold—although the person-on-the-street would have been even more revolted by Harry Lyme's use of the free market in *The Third Man*. Health care was not perceived as a privilege tightly controlled by governmental or medical elites. Weren't physicians supposed to offer aid to the sick and the infirm? Keefer and his Committee, however, represented the "red tape" of bureaucracy—a real barrier to life-saving treatment. Many Americans did not understand that the COC, but one facet of wartime bureaucracy, was simply trying to ration penicillin as equitably as possible.

The sober stance of the COC seemed callous in the face of the patient's suffering. It is difficult to imagine the pain and bewilderment of the family members and patients whom the COC had denied. Having heard so much about the seemingly panacean properties of penicillin, many might have found it difficult to understand a refusal to treat them. Although the hardships of the 1930s prevented many Americans from receiving proper medical care, few had experienced non-economic barriers that prevented their access to treatment. Chester Keefer tested the limits of the professional authority of the American medical practitioners by making physicians "gatekeepers" who guarded access to medical care. By the 1980s, physicians assumed an even greater role in distributional issues as many physicians affiliated themselves with health maintenance organizations or faced decisions about the eligibility of a patient for a donor organ or kidney dialysis.[12]

The distributional questions of wartime penicillin differed little from the issues of the rationing of scarce medical resources several decades later. Although the materials and techniques themselves have changed—donor organs and dialysis have replaced penicillin in the public mind—the crucial issues remain the same. Questions of which patient will receive a donor organ confront contemporary physicians no less than dilemmas of penicillin rationing faced wartime doctors. The ability of medical science to cure serious illness and extend human life may have changed since the Second World War, yet the problem of "Who shall live?" continues to appear in forums that range from *Donahue* to the *New England Journal of Medicine*. The wartime experience of the COC with penicillin represented but a foretaste of the distributional questions that would face the medical community more than forty years later. The penicillin rationing program of the COC, however, also provides late twentieth century policymakers with a viable, practical model for the equitable distribution of scarce medical resources.[13]

Notes

1. See especially John T. Noonan, Jr., *Persons and Masks of the Law: Cardozo, Jefferson, and Wythe as Makers of the Mask* (New York, 1976); see also David Mechanic, "The Growth of Medical Technology and Bureaucracy: Implications for Medical Care," *Milbank Memorial Fund Quarterly* 55 (Winter 1977): 61-78.

2. The most concise discussion of MacNeal, Loewe, and Dawson appears in Gladys Hobby, *Penicillin: Meeting the Challenge* (New Haven, 1985), 165-170.

3. John S. Lockwood to Chester S. Keefer, 12 August 1943, Committee on Medical Research Files, Record Group 227, National Archives, Washington, D.C.; Eleanor Roosevelt to Chester S. Keefer, 24 December 1943; Eleanor Roosevelt to Chester S. Keefer, 29 December 1943; Chester S. Keefer to Eleanor Roosevelt, 30 December 1943, Eleanor Roosevelt Collection, Franklin Delano Roosevelt Library, Hyde Park, N.Y. On cooperative clinical research, see Harry Marks, "Notes from the Underground: The Social Organization of Therapeutic Research, 1920-1950," in Diana Long and Russell Maulitz, eds., *Grand Rounds: One Hundred Years of Internal Medicine* (Philadelphia, 1988), 297-336.

4. Proposal of the Task Committee on Civilian Distribution, 6 April 1944, 2-4, War Production Board Files, Record Group 179, National Archives, Washington, D.C.

5. John Stuart Mill, "Utilitarianism," in Stanley Joel Reiser, Arthur J. Dyck, and William J. Curran, eds., *Ethics in Medicine: Historical Perspectives and Contemporary Concerns* (Cambridge, Mass. 1977), 79-87; Rem B. Edwards and Glenn C. Graber, *Bioethics* (San Diego, 1988), 7-10.

6. James H. Jones, *Bad Blood: The Tuskegee Syphilis Experiment* (New York, 1981).

7. See especially James F. Childress, "Who Shall Live When Not All Can Live?" *Soundings* 53 (Winter 1970): 339-355; Tom L. Beauchamp and James F. Childress, *Principles of Biomedical Ethics* (New York, 1979), 188-200.

8. *Ibid.*

9. *Ibid.*

10. *Ibid.*

11. See especially Barry D. Karl, *The Uneasy State: The United States from 1915 to 1945* (Chicago, 1983), 80-181; Robert H. Wiebe, *The Search for Order: 1877-1920* (New York, 1967).

12. See especially David Mechanic, *From Advocacy to Allocation: The Evolving American Health Care System* (New York, 1986); John C. Burnham, "American Medicine's Golden Age: What Happened to It?" *Science* 215 (19 March 1982): 1474-1475; Chris Cassel, "Doctors and Allocation Decisions: A New Role in the New Medicare," *Journal of Health and Politics* 10 (1985): 549-564; Deborah A. Stone, "Physicians as Gatekeepers: Illness Certification as a Rationing Device," *Public Policy* 27 (Spring 1979): 222-254.

13. See especially Beauchamp and Childress, *Principles of Biomedical Ethics*, esp. 188-200.

Table 3-1

Civilian Penicillin Requests, January 1943 through May 1944

Month	Total
January 1943	0
February 1943	3
March 1943	0
April 1943	2
May 1943	7
June 1943	14
July 1943	13
August 1943	22
September 1943	30
October 1943	25
November 1943	21
December 1943	9
January 1944	10
February 1944	16
March 1944	8
April 1944	5
	185

Note: This sample is based on requests available in the Committee on Medical Research Files, Record Group 227, National Archives, Washington, D.C. From January 1943 through April 1944, 9,750 physicians requested penicillin for the treatment of their patients. The COC released the drug for the treatment of 5,516 cases. It should be noted that this sample of 185 requests, therefore, represents only a fraction of the total number of requests sent to Chester Keefer and the Committee on Chemotherapeutic and Other Agents. (Chester S. Keefer, "Penicillin: A Wartime Accomplishment," in E. C. Andrus, ed., *Advances in Military Medicine*, 721.)

Bibliography

Archival Materials

Boston, Mass. Boston University School of Medicine. Chester S. Keefer Papers.

Hyde Park, N.Y., Franklin Delano Roosevelt Library. Eleanor Roosevelt Collection.

Madison, Wis. Kremers Reference Files, F.B. Power Pharmaceutical Library, University of Wisconsin, Madison.

Suitland, Md. National Archives Annex. Record Group 208. Office of War Information Files.

Washington, D.C. National Academy of Sciences. Division of Medical Sciences, Committees on Military Medicine Files.

Washington, D.C. National Archives. Record Group 108. Motion Picture Archives.

Washington, D.C. National Archives. Record Group 179. War Production Board Files.

Washington, D.C. National Archives. Record Group 227. Committee on Medical Research General Correspondence Files.

Personal Interviews

Anderson, Donald G. Interview with author. Magnolia Springs, Ala., 5 January 1985.

Dowling, Harry F. Interview with author. Cockeysville, Md., 2 May 1986.

Forbes, Thomas R. Interview with Drew F. Amery. New Haven, Conn., 13 August 1986.

MacDonald, Constance Haynes. Interview with author. Boston, Mass., 29 May 1985.

Contemporary Newspaper Articles

"Army to Get Its Magic Penicillin, Needs 5 Billion Units Weekly." *New York Herald-Tribune*, 30 July 1943, 1.

"Making Penicillin in Home Suggested." *New York Times*, 11 November 1943, 24.

"Penicillin." *New York Times*, 19 December 1943, sect. 4, 9.

"Penicillin Is Flown to Girl by the Army." *New York Times*, 5 September 1943, 31.

"Penicillin Saves Child." *New York Times*, 26 September 1943, 28.

"Penicillin Supply Is Far Short of Demand; Army Gets Less than Half, Says Gen. Kirk." *New York Times*, 28 August 1943, 24.

"Set Plans to Rule Penicillin Supply." *New York Times*, 26 August 1943, 52.

Contemporary Magazine Articles

"Cows Need Penicillin, too." *Newsweek*, 3 September 1945, 1.

"Cure by Toothpaste." *Newsweek*, 25 December 1945, 73.

De Kruif, Paul. "Conquest of a Killer." *Reader's Digest*, March 1945, 27-31.

"Doctor Alexander Fleming: His Penicillin Will Save More Lives than War Can Spend." *Time* 15 May 1944, front cover.

"Don't Waste Penicillin." *Science News Letter*, 24 March 1945, 179.

"$5 Penicillin Factory." *Science News Letter*, 4 December 1943, 364-365.

Gardner, Mona. "Miracle from Mold." *Woman's Home Companion*, September 1943, 70.

"How Belts Help Speed the Supply of Precious Penicillin." *Newsweek*, 7 August 1944, 56.

"How Penicillin Is Dried with Frick Refrigeration." *Newsweek*, 11 December 1944, 112.

"New RCA Penicillin Process Speeds Production." *Newsweek*, 6 November 1944, 83.

"Penicillin for All." *Science News Letter*, 27 November 1943, 350.

"Penicillin for Civilians On Sale at Drug Stores." *Science News Letter*, 17 March 1945, 168.

"Penicillin Has Gone to the Dogs." *Newsweek*, 9 July 1945.

"Penicillin in Lozenges." *Science News Letter*, 6 January 1945, 2.

"Penicillin Is 'Shop Talk' to These Rabbits." *Newsweek*, 10 July 1944, 62.

"Penicillin . . . Life Saver." *Newsweek*, 17 April 1944.

"Penicillin's Purity is Guarded by Electronics." *Newsweek*, 28 August 1944, 46.

"Penicillin Use Honored." *New York Times*, 14 January 1944, 9.

"Powder of Life." *Newsweek*, 16 October 1944, 63.

"Public Vies with Army for Penicillin, Miracle Drug that Comes from Mold." *Newsweek*, 30 August 1943, 68.

"Rush on Penicillin." *Time*, 30 August 1943, 44-46.

"Ten for Penicillin." *Newsweek*, 26 March 1945, 93.

"20th Century Seer." *Time*, 15 May 1944, 61-68.

"What'll It Be . . . Wheels or Wings?" *Newsweek*, 3 April 1944, 49.

"What Wonders Do You See in Store for the Postwar Electrical Home ?" *Newsweek*, 30 April 1944, 45.

"Why Did Penicillin Almost Perish?" *Newsweek*, 6 November 1944, 83.

"Why the Army Tells Us that More of Our Boys Will Come Home!" *Newsweek*, 25 December 1944.

"Will Your Post-War House Be a Soap-Bubble?" *Newsweek* 10 April 1944, 97.

"You'll Thrive in This Culture Medium." *Newsweek*, 18 June 1945.

Contemporary Journal Articles

"Abuse of Penicillin." *The New England Journal of Medicine* 233 (27 December 1945): 831.

Bibliography

Anderson, Donald G., and Keefer, Chester S. "Treatment of Non-hemolytic Streptococcus Subacute Bacterial Endocarditis with Penicillin." *Medical Clinics of North America* (September 1945): 1129.

Barker, A. Neish, "Allergic Reactions to Penicillin." *The Lancet* 1 (10 February 1945): 178.

Bruner, Jerome S. "OWI and the American Public." *Public Opinion Quarterly* 7 (Spring 1943): 8.

"Certification of Penicillin and Derivative Drugs." In *Legislative History of the Federal Food, Drug, and Cosmetic Act and Its Amendments*, Vol. 7., n.d., Washington: U.S. Department of Health, Education, and Welfare.

Coghill, Robert D., and Koch, Roy S. "Penicillin—A Wartime Accomplishment." *Chemical and Engineering News* 23 (1946): 2310-2316.

Dailey, Donald. "What Will the Postwar Consumer Want?" *Advertising and Selling*, June 1943, 54.

Davis, Elmer. "The OWI Has a Job." *Public Opinion Quarterly* 7 (Spring 1943): 8.

Elder, Albert L., and Monroe, Lawrence A. "Penicillin: Wartime Growing Pains of the Industry." *Chemical and Metallurgical Engineering* 51 (March 1944): 103-105.

Falk, Leslie. "Is the Indiscriminate Use of Penicillin Imminent?" *Journal of the American Pharmaceutical Association* 34 (1945): 126-127.

_____. "Will Penicillin Be Used Indiscriminately?" *New England Journal of Medicine* 127 (17 March 1945): 672.

Felsenfeld, Oscar. "Yeast-like Fungi in the Intestinal Tract of Chronically Institutionalized Patients," *American Journal of Medical Science* 207 (January 1944): 60-62.

Fichelis, Robert P. "Penicillin: Opportunity and Obligation." *Journal of the American Pharmaceutical Association* 6 (April 1945): 91-92.

Fielding, Robert S., and Queen, Frank B. "Strain Variations in Penicillin Sensitivity Among Bacterial Species Encountered in War Wounds and Infections." *American Journal of Clinical Pathology* 16 (1946): 63.

Filsinger, Frederick W. "The Forgotten People," *Hospital Management* 56 (November 1943): 20-21.

Hamblin, Terry. "Personal View." *British Medical Journal* (10 August 1974): 407.

Hamilton, Paul M. "Some Points on the Control of Penicillin When It Is Sent to Hospitals," *Hospitals* 18 (May 1944): 62.

Hamre, Dorothy M.; Rake, Geoffrey; McKee, Clara, M.; and MacPhillamy, Harold B. "The Toxicity of Penicillin as Prepared for Clinical Use," *American Journal of Medical Science* 206 (November 1943): 642-652.

Harley, H.R.S.; Baty, J.A.; and Bowie, J.H. "The Pathogenicity of Penicillin-Insensitive Infection," *British Medical Journal* 1 (27 April 1946): 639-643.

Hewlett, Albion Walter. "Eight Years in the Department of Internal Medicine." *Transactions of the Clinical Society of the University of Michigan* 7 (1916): 146-149.

Jetter, Walter W., and Hadley, Rollin V. "A Study of Casualties in Institutions under the Supervision of the Massachusetts

Department of Health." *American Journal of Psychiatry* 100 (January 1944): 515.

Kaufman, Paul. "Prophylactic Effect of Pneumococcus Polysaccharide Against Pneumonia," *Archives of Internal Medicine* 61 (1941): 304-319.

Keefer, Chester Scott. "Official Statement Concerning Streptomycin." *Journal of the American Medical Association* 131 (4 May 1946): 131.

_____. "Penicillin—Its Present Status in the Treatment of Infections." *American Journal of Medical Science* 210 (August 1945): 155.

_____. "Penicillin: A Wartime Accomplishment." In *Advances in Military Medicine Made by American Investigators Working Under the Sponsorship of the Committee on Medical Research*, vol. II, edited by E.C. Andrus. Boston: Little, Brown, and Co., 1948.

_____. "Streptomycin in the Treatment of Infections." *Journal of the American Medical Association* 132 (7 September 1946): 4-5.

_____. "Streptomycin in the Treatment of Infections." *Journal of the American Medical Association* 132 (14 September 1946): 74-77.

_____; Blake, Francis G.; Marshall, E.K., Jr.; Lockwood, John S.; and Wood, W. Barry, Jr. "Penicillin in the Treatment of Infections." *Journal of the American Medical Association* 122 (28 August 1943): 1217-1224.

Larkey, Sanford V. "The National Research Council and Medical Preparedness." *War Medicine* 1 (January 1941): 70-79.

O'Leary, Paul M. "Wartime Rationing and Government Organization." *American Political Science Review* 34 (December 1945): 1089.

Peabody, Francis W. "The Department of Medicine at the Peking Union Medical College." *Science* 56 (22 September 1922): 317-320.

"Penicillin." *American Professional Pharmacist* 10 (May 1944): 315.

"Penicillin." *American Professional Pharmacist* 10 (July 1944): 465.

"Penicillin Comes to the Corner Pharmacy." *Journal of the American Pharmaceutical Association* 6 (April 1945): 90.

"Penicillin for Civilians Ready Soon; Plan Distribution Through Hospitals." *Hospitals* 19 (May 1944): 82.

"Penicillin Sodium." *American Professional Pharmacist* 10 (August 1944): 539.

"Pretesting and Certification of Streptomycin." In *Legislative History of the Federal Food, Drug, and Cosmetic Act and Its Amendments*, Vol. 7. Washington: U.S. Department of Health, Education, and Welfare.

Raper, Kenneth B. and Coghill, Robert D. " 'Home Made' Penicillin." *Journal of the American Medical Association* 123 (25 December 1943): 1135.

Richards, A.N. "The Impact of the War on Medicine." *Science* 103 (10 May 1946): 578.

_____. "Penicillin: Statement Released by Committee on Medical Research." *Journal of the American Medical Association* 122 (22 May 1943): 235-236.

Robinson, Harry J. "Toxicity and Efficacy of Penicillin." *Journal of Pharmacology and Experimental Therapeutics* 77 (January 1943): 70-79.

Rostenberg, Adolph, Jr., and Welch, Henry. "A Study of the Types of Hypersensitivity Induced by Penicillin." *American Journal of Medical Science* 210 (August 1945): 167.

Weiss, Soma. "Self-Observations and Psychologic Reactions of Medical Student A.S.R. to the Onset and Symptoms of Subacute Bacterial Endocarditis." *Journal of the Mount Sinai Hospital* (1941-1942): 1079-1094.

"What of the Morrow?" *American Professional Pharmacist* 10 (September 1944): 619.

Woodman, Robert. "There Is Room for Improvement in Our Mental Disease Hospitals: Facts and Figures on These Public Hospitals—What to Do About Them." *Modern Hospital* 61 (November 1943): 78.

Contemporary Books

Anderson, Donald G., and Keefer, Chester S. *The Therapeutic Value of Penicillin: A Study of 10,000 Cases.* Ann Arbor, Mich.: J.W. Edwards, 1948.

Andrus, E.C., et al., eds. *Advances in Military Medicine Made by American Investigators Working Under the Sponsorship of the Committee on Medical Research*, 2 vols. Office of Scientific Research and Development, Science in World War II Series. Boston: Little, Brown, and Co., 1948.

Baxter, Jr., James Phinney. *Scientists Against Time.* Boston: Little, Brown and Co., 1946.

Blumgarten, A.S. *Textbook of Materia Medica*. 5th edition, revised. New York: MacMillan, 1931.

Boas, Ernst P. *Treatment of the Patient Past Fifty*. Chicago: Yearbook Publishers, 1941.

Bush, Vannevar. *Science, The Endless Frontier*. Washington, D.C.: U. S. Government Printing Office, 1945.

Chapin, F. Stuart. *The Impact of the War on Community Leadership and Opinion in Red Wing*. Community Basis for Postwar Planning Series, No. 3, April 1945. Minneapolis: University of Minnesota Press, 1945.

De Kruif, Paul. *Life Among the Doctors*. New York: Harcourt, Brace, and Co., 1949.

_____. *Microbe Hunters*. New York: Harcourt, Brace, and Co., 1926.

Fishbein, Morris, ed. *Doctors at War*. New York: E.P. Dutton, 1945.

Gallup, George H. *The Gallup Poll: Public Opinion, 1935-1971*, 2 vols. New York: Random House, 1972.

Greene, Graham. *The Third Man and the Fallen Idol*. London: Heinemann, 1964.

Lewis, Sinclair. *Arrowsmith*. New York: Harcourt, Brace and World, 1925.

Musser, John H., ed. *Internal Medicine: Its Theory and Practice in Contributions by American Authors* 2d rev. ed. Philadelphia: Lea and Feibiger, 1934.

Ratcliff, J.D. *Yellow Magic: The Story of Penicillin.* New York: Random House, 1945.

Stewart, Irvin. *Organizing Scientific Research for War: The Administrative History of the Office of Scientific Research and Development.* Office of Scientific Research and Development, Science in World War II Series. Boston: Little, Brown, and Co., 1948.

Sullivan, Lawrence. *The Dead Hand of Bureaucracy.* Indianapolis, Ind.: Bobbs-Merrill, 1940.

Wriston, Henry M. *Challenge to Freedom.* New York: Harper and Brothers, 1943.

Zinsser, Hans, and Bayne-Jones, Stanhope. *A Textbook of Bacteriology*, 8th ed., revised. New York: Appleton-Century, 1939.

Other Works

Articles

Adams, David P. "The Penicillin Mystique and the Popular Press (1935-1950)." *Pharmacy in History* 26 (1984): 134-142.

––––––––. "Wartime Bureaucracy and Penicillin Allocation: The Committee on Chemotherapeutic and Other Agents, 1942-1944." *Journal of the History of Medicine and Allied Sciences* 44 (April 1989): 196-217.

Annas, George. "Life, Liberty, and the Pursuit of Organ Sales." *The Hastings Center Report* 14 (February 1984): 22-23.

Auerbach, Lewis. "Scientists in the New Deal: A Pre-War Episode in the Relations Between Science and Government in the United States." *Minerva* (1965): 457-482.

Austin, J. Harold. "A Brief Sketch of the History of the American Society for Clinical Investigation." *Journal of Clinical Investigation* 28 (1949): 401-408.

Austrian, Robert. "Perrin Hamilton Long, 1899-1965." *Transactions of the Association of American Physicians* 79 (1966): 59-61.

Avorn, Jerry; Chen, Milton; and Hartley, Robert. "Scientific versus Commercial Sources of Influence on the Prescribing Behavior of Physicians." *American Journal of Medicine* 73 (July 1982): 4-8.

J. B. "Organs for Sale: From Marketplace to Jungle." *The Hastings Center Report* 16 (February 1986): 3-4.

Baily, Mary Ann. " 'Rationing' and American Health Policy." *Journal of Health Politics, Policy and Law* 9 (Fall 1984): 489-501.

Basson, Marc D. "Choosing Among Candidates for Scarce Medical Resources." *Journal of Medicine and Philosophy* 4 (1979): 313-333.

Blumstein, James F. "Rationing Medical Resources: A Constitutional, Legal, and Policy Analysis." *Texas Law Review* 59 (November 1981): 1345-1399.

Brainard, Ellen R. "History of the American Society for Clinical Investigation, 1909-1959." *Journal of Clinical Investigation* 38 (1959): 1784-1818.

Brown, Ethan Allan. "Reactions to Penicillin: A Review of the Literature, 1943-1948." *Annals of Allergy* 6 (November-December 1948): 723-746.

Burnham, John C. "American Medicine's Golden Age: What Happened to It?" *Science* 215 (19 March 1982): 1474-1475.

Cassel, Chris. "Doctors and Allocation Decisions: A New Role in the New Medicare." *Journal of Health Politics, Policy and Law* 10 (1985): 549-564.

Castorina, Edward. "Scarce Life-Saving Medical Resources: Equal Protection and Patient Selection." *Journal of Legal Medicine* 1 (July 1979): 154-185.

Childress, James F. "Who Shall Live When Not All Can Live?" *Soundings* 53 (Winter 1970): 339-355.

Cranford, Ronald E., and Doudera, A. Edward. "The Emergence of Institutional Ethics Committees." *Law, Medicine, and Health Care* (February 1984): 13-20.

D'Amelio, Nea. "Are Family Doctors Prescribing Too Many Antibiotics?" *Medical Times* 102 (January 1974): 53-61.

──────. "What Young Doctors Told Us About Antibiotic Overkill." *Medical Times* (March 1974): 144-153.

Doolen, Richard M. "The Founding of the University of Michigan Hospital: An Innovation in Medical Education." *Journal of Medical Education* 39 (1964): 50-57.

Dowling, Harry F. "The Effect of the Emergence of Resistant Strains on the Future of Antibiotic Therapy." *Antibiotics Annual* (1953-1954): 27-34.

──────. "The History of Broad Spectrum Antibiotics." *Antibiotics Annual* (1958-1959): 39-44.

Elliot, Clark A. "Models of the American Scientist: A Look at Collective Biography." *Isis* 73 (1982): 79-89.

Endicott, Kenneth M., and Allen, Ernest M. "The Growth of Medical Research 1941-1953 and the Role of the Public

Health Service Research Grants." *Science* 118 (25 September 1953): 341.

"Fund Is Established for Girl with Five Transplanted Organs." *New York Times* (29 December 1987), 11.

Finer, Herman. "Critics of 'Bureaucracy'." *Political Science Quarterly* 60 (March 1945): 100-112.

Garrod, Lawrence P. Letter to the Editor. *British Medical Journal* (28 September 1974): 805.

Hamblin, Terry. "Personal View." *British Medical Journal* (10 August 1974): 407.

Hare, Ronald, "The Scientific Discoveries of Alexander Fleming Other than the Discovery of Penicillin." *Medical History* 27 (1983): 347-372.

Hastings, A. Baird. "Chester Scott Keefer, M.D., D.Sc.: Physician and Teacher Extraordinary." *The Boston Medical Quarterly* 14 (September 1963): 89-90.

Hewetson, Debra S. "Scarce Medical Resource Allocation—The Case of First Impression: A Hypothetical Opinion of the Twelfth Circuit United States Court of Appeals." *Journal of Legal Medicine* 3 (1982): 295-315.

Hey, C. V. Letter to the Editor. *British Medical Journal* (28 September 1974): 805.

Hirsch, James G. "William Barry Wood, Jr.: May 4, 1910–March 9, 1971." *Biographical Memoirs of the National Academy of Sciences* (1979): 387-418.

Hussar, Allen E. "A Proposed Crusade for the Rational Use of Antibiotics." *Antibiotics Annual* (1954-1955): 379-381.

Jones, Kenneth MacDonald, "The Endless Frontier." *Prologue* 8 (Spring 1976): 35-46.

Jones, Philip N.; Bigham, Roy S.; and Manning, Phil R. "Use of Antibiotics in Nonbacterial Respiratory Infections." *Journal of the American Medical Association* 153 (26 September 1953): 262-264.

Kargon, Robert, and Hodes, Elizabeth. "Karl Compton, Isaiah Bowman, and the Politics of Science in the Great Depression." *Isis* 76 (September 1985): 301-318.

Karl, Barry D. "Philanthropy, Policy Planning, and the Bureaucratization of the Democratic Ideal." *Daedalus* (Summer 1975): 129-149.

Kolata, Gina. "Imminent Marketing of AZT Raises Problems." *Science* 235 (20 March 1987): 1462-1463.

Lewin, Tamar. "Mother Sued Over Payment for Son's Liver Transplants." *New York Times* (11 November 1984), sec. A, 24.

Long, Perrin H. "Fatal Anaphylactic Reactions to Penicillin." *Antibiotics Annual* (1953-1954): 35-40.

Maren, Thomas H. "Eli Kennerly Marshall, Jr., 1889-1966." *Bulletin of the Johns Hopkins Hospital* 119 (October 1966): 246-254.

Massell, Benedict F., et al. "Penicillin and the Marked Decrease in Morbidity and Mortality from Rheumatic Fever in the United States." *New England Journal of Medicine* 318 (4 February 1988): 280-286.

Mechanic, David M. "The Growth of Medical Technology and Bureaucracy: Implications for Medical Care." *Milbank Memorial Fund Quarterly* 55 (Winter 1977): 61-78.

———. "How Should Medical Care Be Rationed?" *American Journal of Medicine* 66 (January 1979): 8-9.

"Organ Transplants: Preference for the Wealthy." *The Lancet* 1 (22 February 1986): 433-434.

Paul, John R. "Francis Gilman Blake, 1888 [*sic*]-1952." *Transactions of the Association of American Physicians* 65 (1952): 9-13.

———. "Francis Gilman Blake: 1887-1952." *Biographical Memoirs of the National Academy of Sciences* (1954): 1-29.

Pellegrino, Edmund D. "Rationing Health Care: The Ethics of Medical Gatekeeping." *Journal of Contemporary Health Law and Policy* 2 (1986): 23-45.

Rapaport, Felix T. "A Rational Approach to a Common Goal: The Equitable Distribution of Organs for Transplantation." *Journal of the American Medical Association* 257 (12 June 1987): 3118-3119.

Raper, Kenneth B. "A Decade of Antibiotics in America." *Mycologia* 44 (January-February 1952): 15.

Rogers, David E. "The Early Years: The Medical World in Which Walsh McDermott Trained." *Daedalus* 115 (Spring 1986): 1-18.

Roland, Alex. "Science and War." *Osiris*, 2d series 1 (1985): 247-272.

Rosenthal, Abraham. "Follow-Up Study of Fatal Penicillin Reactions." *Journal of the American Medical Association* 167 (28 June 1958): 1118-1121.

Rossiter, Margaret. "Science and Public Policy since World War II." *Osiris*, 2nd series, 1 (1985): 273-294.

Sanford, Fillmore H. "Public Orientation to Roosevelt." *Public Opinion Quarterly* 15 (Summer 1951): 189-215.

Schlegel, Robert J. "The Formulation of Health Policy." In *Biomedical Scientists and Public Policy*, edited by H. Hugh Fudenberg and Vijaya L. Melnick. New York: Plenum Press, 1978.

Simmons, Henry E., and Stolley, Paul D. "This Is Medical Progress? Trends and Consequences of Antibiotic Use in the United States." *Journal of the American Medical Association* 227 (4 March 1974): 1023-1028.

Spears, Jack. "The Doctor on the Screen." *Films in Review* 6 (1955): 436-444.

Stone, Deborah A. "Physicians as Gatekeepers: Illness Certification as a Rationing Device." *Public Policy* 27 (Spring 1979): 227-254.

Sussman, Leila A. "FDR and the White House Mail." *Public Opinion Quarterly* 20 (Spring 1956): 5-6.

Swann, John Patrick. "The Search for Penicillin Synthesis during World War II." *British Journal for the History of Science* 16 (July 1983): 154-190.

Teigen, Philip M. "William Osler as Medical Hero." *Bulletin of the History of Medicine* 60 (Winter 1986): 573-576.

Tillett, W.S. "Perrin Hamilton Long, 1889-1966." *Transactions of the Association of American Physicians* 79 (1966): 59.

Trent, Bill. "Is Media Hype Necessary for Organ Transplants?" *Canadian Medical Association Journal* 130 (15 March 1984): 774-780.

"A Verray Parfit Praktisour [*sic*]." *Medical Times* 94 (June 1966): 686-702.

Wainwright, Milton, and Swan, Harold T. "C.G. Paine and the Earliest Surviving Clinical Records of Penicillin Therapy." *Medical History* 30 (1986): 42-56.

Wallis, Claudia. "Of Television and Transplants." *Time* (23 June 1986), 68.

Wilkins, Robert W. "Chester Scott Keefer: 1897-1972." *Transactions of the Association of American Physicians* 85 (1972): 24-26.

Books

Aaron, Henry J., and Schwartz, William B., *The Painful Prescription: Rationing Hospital Care*. Studies in Social Economics Series. Washington, D.C.: Brookings Institution, 1984.

Beauchamp, Tom L., and Childress, James F. *Principles of Biomedical Ethics*. New York: Oxford University Press, 1979.

Becker, Howard S; Geer, Blanche; Hughes, Everett C.; and Strauss, Anselm L. *Boys in White: Student Culture in Medical School*. Chicago: University of Chicago Press, 1961.

Beecher, Henry K., and Altschule, Mark D. *Medicine at Harvard: The First Three Hundred Years*. Hanover, N.H.: University Press of New England, 1977.

Berliner, Howard S. *A System of Scientific Medicine: Philanthropic Foundations in the Flexner Era*. New York: Methuen, 1985.

Blank, Robert. *Rationing Medicine*. New York: Columbia University Press, 1988.

Bliss, Michael. *The Discovery of Insulin*. Chicago: University of Chicago Press, 1982.

Blum, John Morton. *V Was for Victory: Politics and Culture during World War II*. New York: Harcourt Brace, 1976.

Bowers, John Z. *Western Medicine in a Chinese Palace: Peking Union Medical College, 1917-1951*. Philadelphia: Josiah Macy, Jr., Foundation, 1972.

Brandt, Allen M. *No Magic Bullet: A Social History of Venereal Disease in the United States since 1880*. New York: Oxford University Press, 1985.

Brown, E. Richard. *Rockefeller Medicine Men: Medicine and Capitalism in America*. Berkeley, Calif.: University of California Press, 1979.

Burns, James M. *Roosevelt: The Soldier of Freedom*. New York: Harcourt, Brace, and Jovanovich, 1970.

Cattell, Jacques, ed. *American Men of Science: A Biographical Directory*. Lancaster, Penn., 1949.

Chesney, Alan M. *The Johns Hopkins Hospital and The Johns Hopkins University School of Medicine: A Chronicle, 1905-1914*. vol III. Baltimore: Johns Hopkins University Press, 1963.

Corner, George W. *A History of the Rockefeller Institute: Origins and Growth, 1901-1953*. New York: Rockefeller Institute Press, 1964.

Cranford, Ronald E., and Doudera, A. Edward, eds. *Institutional Ethics Committees and Health Care Decision Making*. Ann Arbor, Mich.: Health Administration Press, 1984.

Dallek, Robert. *Franklin D. Roosevelt and American Foreign Policy, 1932-1945*. New York: Oxford University Press, 1979.

Daniels, Roger. *Concentration Camps USA: Japanese Americans and World War II*. New York: Holt, Rinehart, and Winston, 1972.

Dowling, Harry F. *City Hospitals: The Undercare of the Underprivileged*. Cambridge, Mass.: Harvard University Press, 1982.

———. *Fighting Infection: Conquests of the Twentieth Century*. Cambridge, Mass.: Harvard University Press, 1977.

Dreiszinger, N.F., ed. *Mobilization for Total War: The Canadian, American and British Experience: 1914-1918, 1939-1945*. Waterloo, Ontario: Wilfred Laurier University Press, 1981.

Duffy, J.C. *Emotional Issues in the Lives of Physicians*. Springfield, Ill.: C. Thomas Press, 1970.

Dupree, A. Hunter. *Science in the Federal Government: A History of Policies and Activities to 1940*. New York: Harper and Row, 1957.

Edwards, Rem B., and Graber, Glenn C. *Bioethics*. San Diego: Harcourt, Brace, and Jovanovich, 1987.

Ferguson, Mary E. *China Medical Board and Peking Union Medical College: A Chronicle of Fruitful Collaboration, 1914-1951*. New York: China Medical Board of New York, 1970.

Fox, Daniel M. *Health Policies, Health Politics: The British and American Experience, 1911-1965*. Princeton: Princeton University Press, 1986.

Fox, Frank W. *Madison Avenue Goes to War: The Strange Military Career of American Advertising*. Charles E. Merrill Monograph Series in the Humanities and Social Sciences, 1. Provo, Utah, 1975.

Freidson, Eliot. *Profession of Medicine: A Study of the Sociology of Applied Knowledge*. New York: Dodd, Mead, and Co., 1970.

_____. *Professional Powers: A Study of the Institutionalization of Formal Knowledge*. Chicago: University of Chicago Press, 1986.

Fuchs, Victor R. *Who Shall Live? Health, Economics, and Social Choice*. New York: Basic Books, 1984.

Fudenberg, H. Hugh, and Melnick, Vijaya L., eds. *Biomedical Scientists and Public Policy*. New York: Plenum Press, 1978.

Goldman, Eric F. *The Crucial Decade and After: 1945-1960*. New York: Vintage Books, 1960.

Greenberg, Daniel S. *The Politics of Pure Science*. New York: New American Library, 1967.

Grusky, Oscar, and Miller, George A., eds. *The Sociology of Organizations: Basic Studies*. New York: Free Press, 1970.

Harden, Victoria A. *Inventing the NIH: Federal Biomedical Research Policy, 1887-1937*. Baltimore: Johns Hopkins University Press, 1986.

Harvey, A. McGehee. *The Interurban Clinical Club (1905-1976): A Record of Achievement in Clinical Science*. Philadelphia: W.B. Saunders, 1978.

———. *Science at the Bedside: Clinical Research in American Medicine, 1905-1945*. Baltimore: Johns Hopkins University Press, 1981.

Haskell, Thomas L., ed. *The Authority of Experts: Studies in History and Theory*. Bloomington, Ind.: Indiana University Press, 1984.

Hobby, Gladys L. *Penicillin: Meeting the Challenge*. New Haven: Yale University Press, 1985.

Honey, Maureen. *Creating Rosie the Riveter: Class, Gender, and Propaganda During World War II*. Amherst: University of Massachusetts Press, 1984.

Irons, Peter H. *The New Deal Lawyers*. Princeton, N.J.: Princeton University Press, 1982.

Jones, James H. *Bad Blood: The Tuskegee Syphilis Experiment*. New York: Free Press, 1981.

Karl, Barry D. *The Uneasy State: The United States, 1915-1945*. Chicago: University of Chicago Press, 1984.

Kaufman, Martin; Galishoff, Stuart; and Savitt, Todd L., eds. *Dictionary of American Medical Biography*, 2 Vols. Westport, Conn.: Greenwood Press, 1984.

Kauper, Paul G., and Beytagh, Francis X. *Constitutional Law: Cases and Materials*, 5th ed. Boston: Little, Brown, and Co., 1980.

Keefer, Chester S. *Medical Science and Society*. Boston: Boston University Press, 1956.

Kevles, Daniel J. *The Physicists: The History of a Scientific Community in Modern America*. New York: Vintage Books, 1977.

Larson, Magali Sarfatti. *The Rise of Professionalism: A Sociological Analysis*. Berkeley: University of California Press, 1977.

Leuchtenberg, William E. *Franklin D. Roosevelt and the New Deal*. New York: Harper and Row, 1963.

Lingeman, Richard. *Don't You Know There's a War On?* New York: Capricorn Books, 1972.

Long, Diana, and Maulitz, Russell, eds. *Grand Rounds: One Hundred Years of Internal Medicine*. Philadelphia: University of Pennsylvania Press, 1988.

Ludmerer, Kenneth M. *Learning to Heal: The Development of American Medical Education*. New York: Basic Books, 1985.

MacFarlane, Gwyn. *Alexander Fleming: The Man and the Myth*. Cambridge, Mass.: Harvard University Press, 1984.

Mechanic, David. *From Advocacy to Allocation: The Evolving American Health Care System*. New York: Free Press, 1986.

Murphy, Paul L. *The Constitution in Crisis Times, 1918-1969*. New York: Harper and Row, 1972.

Nelson, William E. *The Roots of American Bureaucracy, 1830-1900*. Cambridge, Mass.: Harvard University Press, 1982.

Noonan, John T., Jr. *Persons and Masks of the Law: Cardozo, Jefferson, and Wythe as Makers of the Masks*. New York: Farrar, Straus, and Giroux, 1976.

Parascandola, John, ed. *The History of Antibiotics: A Symposium*. Madison, Wis.: American Institute for the History of Pharmacy, 1980.

Patterson, James T. *The Dread Disease: Cancer and Modern American Culture*. Cambridge, Mass.: Harvard University Press, 1987.

Pennick, James L., Jr.; Pursell, Carroll W., Jr.; Sherwood, Morgan B.; Swain, Donald C., eds. *The Politics of American Science, 1939 to the Present*. Chicago: Rand McNally, 1965.

Perrett, Geoffrey. *Days of Sadness, Years of Triumph: The American People, 1939-1945*. New York: Coward, McCann and Geohegan, 1973.

Phibbs, Brendan, *The Other Side of Time: A Combat Surgeon in World War II*. Boston: Little, Brown, and Co., 1987.

Polenberg, Richard. *War and Society in the United States: 1941-1945*. New York: Lippincott, 1972.

Reiser, Stanley Joel; Dyck, Arthur J.; and Curran, William J. eds. *Ethics in Medicine: Historical Perspectives and Contemporary Concerns*. Cambridge, Mass.: MIT Press, 1977.

Rosen, Eliot A. *Hoover, Roosevelt, and the Brains Trust: From Depression to New Deal*. New York: Columbia University Press, 1977.

Rosen, George. *The Structure of American Medical Practice, 1875-1941*, ed. by Charles E. Rosenberg. Philadelphia: University of Pennsylvania Press, 1983.

Rosenberg, Charles E. *No Other Gods: On Science and American Social Thought*. Baltimore: Johns Hopkins University Press, 1976.

Schlesinger, Arthur, Jr. *The Age of Roosevelt: The Crisis of the Old Order*. Boston: Houghton and Mifflin, 1957.

Sheehan, John C. *The Enchanted Ring: The Untold Story of Penicillin*. Cambridge, Mass.: MIT Press, 1982.

Shryock, Richard H. *American Medical Research: Past and Present*. New York: Commonwealth Fund, 1947.

Smith, Lawrence Weld, and Walker, Ann Dolan. *Penicillin Decade, 1941-1951: Sensitizations and Toxicities*. Washington, D.C.: Arundel Press, 1951.

Sokoloff, Boris. *The Miracle Drugs*. Chicago: Yearbook Publishers, 1949.

Spink, Wesley W. *Infectious Diseases: Prevention and Treatment in the Nineteenth and Twentieth Centuries*. Minneapolis: University of Minnesota Press, 1978.

Starr, Paul. *The Social Transformation of American Medicine*. New York: Basic Books, 1982.

Stevens, Rosemary. *American Medicine and the Public Interest*. New Haven: Yale University Press, 1972.

Strickland, Stephen P. *Politics, Science and Dread Disease: A Short History of United States Medical Research*. Cambridge, Mass.: Harvard University Press, 1972.

Temin, Peter. *Taking Your Medicine: Drug Regulation in the United States*. Cambridge, Mass.: Harvard University Press, 1980.

Tobey, Ronald C. *The American Ideology of National Science, 1919-1930*. Pittsburgh: University of Pittsburgh Press, 1971.

Tugwell, R.G. *The Brains Trust*. New York: Viking Press, 1968.

Tyor, Peter L., and Bell, Leland V. *Caring for the Retarded in America: A History*, Contributions in Medical History, Number 15. Westport, Conn.: Greenwood Press, 1984.

Vaughn, Stephen. *Holding Fast the Inner Lines: Democracy, Nationalism, and the Committee on Public Information*. Chapel Hill: University of North Carolina Press, 1980.

Veysey, Laurence R. *The Emergence of the American University*. Chicago: University of Chicago Press, 1965.

Vogel, Morris J. *The Invention of the Modern Hospital: Boston, 1870-1930*. Chicago: University of Chicago Press, 1980.

Welch, Henry, and Marti-Ibanez, Felix. *The Antibiotic Saga*. New York: Yearbook Publishers, 1960.

Wiebe, Robert H. *The Search for Order: 1877-1920*. New York: Hill and Wang, 1967.

Winkler, Allan M. *The Politics of Propaganda: The Office of War Information, 1942-1945*. New Haven, Conn.: Yale University Press, 1978.

Winslow, Gerald R. *Triage and Justice*. Berkeley: University of California Press, 1982.

Wynn, Neil A. *The Afro-American and the Second World War*. New York: Holmes and Meier, 1976.

Index

A

Abbott Pharmeceuticals, 38, 82-83
Academeic physicians, 45-59, 158, 162-173
    books about, 56-57
    motion pictures about, 56-58
Advertisements, 118-121, 123
AIDS, 175
Alcoholics, 186
Alexander, E. L., 110
Allen, Ernest M., 164, 166
Allergies
    anaphylactic shock, 161
    to penicillin, 155-157, 159, 161
    Staphylococcus aureus superinfections, 171
    to streptomycin, 171
    unticaria, 161, 171
Amebiasis, 173
American Medical Association (AMA), 57, 92, 135, 161
American Society for Clinical Investigation (ASCI), 30, 45, 51-54
American Society of Bacteriologists, 82
Ampicillin, 173
Anaphylactic shock, 161
Anderson, Donald, 70, 86-87, 93, 154, 156, 167-168
Anderson, George K., 68-69
Andrus, E. C., 74, 88, 104
Appeals Board, 173
Armed Forces Epidemiological Board, 167
Aureomycin, 168, 173, 176
Ayer, H. W., 120
AZT, 5, 18, 158, 175

B

Baby Jesse, 2-3
Bacteremia, 170

Bacterial endocarditis, 98, 113, 142, 159, 185-186
    subacute bacterial endocarditis (SBE), 15-16, 78-81, 189
Baily, Mary Ann, 1-2
Baird, William F., 110
Balfour, Donald, 85
Banting, Frederick, 11-12, 14
Barker, E. Tefft, 71-73, 80-81
Barker, Marie, 75-76, 80, 93, 96, 113
Barnes Hospital, 32, 47, 50
Basson, Marc D., 11
Baxter, James Phinney, 56
Bell, Leland, 137
Best, Charles, 11
Billings, John Shaw, 47
Blackmarket, 131, 133, 144-146
Blake, Francis G., 27, 31-32, 51-54, 80, 167
Blank, Robert, 3
Bliss, Eleanor, 28, 50, 104
Bliss, Michael, 12
Blumstein, James F., 67
Boas, Ernst, 136
Bone marrow transplants, 3
Books, 144-145
Boston City Hospital (BCH), 32, 48, 50, 52
Boston University School of Medicine, 32, 70, 167-168
Bowers, John Z., 52
Brooklyn Jewish Hospital, 15
Brucellosis, 171, 173
Burnham, John C., 57, 161
Burroughs Wellcome, 175
Bush, Vannevar, 65-66, 84, 117, 132, 162-166
Bushnell Hospital, 35-38, 51, 69, 105

C

Cancer, 70, 88, 144, 166

National Cancer Institute (NCI), 165, 167
Caplan, Arthur, 4
Cardiovascular disease, 166
Carraway, Hattie, 87
Carter, Anne Shirley, 106
Cartoons, 117-118
Chemicals Bureau, 138
Cholramphenicol, 168, 173-174, 176
Clarke, Hans T., 122
Clostridial infections, 8, 35
Coghill, Robert, 114-115, 117, 121, 123, 168
Colds, 174
Colitis, 90-91, 186
Columbia-Presbyterian Hospital, 8, 47, 51
Columbia University's College of Physicians and Surgeons, 15, 29, 47, 51, 55, 167
Commercial Solvents Corporation, 118-119, 121
Committee on Chemotherapeutic and Other Agents (COC), 5-7, 10-17, 25-39, 45, 66-93, 103-104, 111, 115, 122-123, 131-134, 143-144, 146, 153, 164, 167, 169-176, 185-190, 193
  members of, 49-61
  Subcommittee on Infectious Diseases, 31-32
  Subcommittee on Surgical Infections, 36, 51
Committee on Public Information, 13, 106
Committee on Transfusions, 26

D

Dame, Lawrence, 104
Davis, Elmer, 16, 116
Davison, W. C., 68
Dawson, Martin Henry, 16, 29-31, 54, 78-79, 85, 185
de Kruif, Paul, 15, 57
Department of Agriculture, 8, 108, 163

Northern Regional Research Laboratory (NRRL), 33, 114, 132
Department of Health, Education, and Welfare, 167
De Silliers, Ronnie, 3-4
Detail men, 158
Dialysis, 3, 18, 145, 190
Division of Medical Sciences (DMS), 6, 25-29, 31, 39, 68, 88, 122
  Committee on Chemotherapeutic and Other Agents (COC), 5-7, 10-17, 25-39, 45, 49-61, 66-93, 103-104, 111, 115, 122-123, 131-134, 143-144, 146, 153, 155, 164, 167, 169-176, 185-190, 193
  Committee on Transfussions, 26
Dock, George, 48
Donahue, Phil, 3, 190
Donor organs, 2-5, 18, 153-154, 190
  legal aspects of, 66-67
  market for, 4-5
Dowling, Harry, 158
Druggists, 140-143
Dupree, A. Hunter, 6-7, 26

E

Elderly, 135-136, 146, 186
Eli Lilly Company, 132
Eliot, Alexander, 115-116
Endicott, Kenneth M., 164, 166
Evans Memorial Hospital, 109

F

Falk, Leslie, 157
Federal Trade Commission, 143, 148
Federal Trade Commission Act, 132
Fichelis, Robert, 134
First World War, 11-13
  Committee on Public Information, 13, 106
  Division of Medical Sciences (DMS), 25

Index

Fishbein, Morris, 38
Fitzgerald, William, 86-87
Fleming, Alexander, 7, 122, 157, 160
Flexner, Simon, 53
Flexner Report, 47
Florey, Howard, 7-8, 29, 122
Food and Drug Administration, 155, 167
Food, Drug, and Cosmetic Act of 1938, 158
Foster, Tabatha, 4
Fourteenth Amendment, 66
Fraser, Ian, 107
Free market distribution, 1-5
   of donor organs, 4-5
   media coverage, 2-3, 5
   of penicillin, 142-146
Fuel Administration, 13
Fulton, John, 122

G
Gardner, Mona, 107
Glaucoma, 70, 88
Goldman, Eric F., 160-161
Goldsmith, Kathleen, 117
Gonorrhea, 86-87, 106, 144
Gore, Albert, 3
Gorham, L. W., 79, 186
Grady Hospital, 114
Gram-negative infections, 170
Great Depression, 13
Greene, Graham, 2, 144

H
Hadassah University Hospital, 106
Hallock, Duncan, 90-91, 186
Hallock, Wilton, 90-91
Harrison, Ross, 85
Harvard Medical School, 15, 32, 47-48, 50-51, 54-55, 79
Harvey, A. McGehee, 48-49, 53
Hastings, A. Baird, 36
Hazel, George, 83
Heatley, Norman G., 8, 132
Hemophilus influenzae infections, 170

Herrell, Wallace, 82-85, 186
Hewetson, Debras S. 66
Higgins, Norris, 86, 93
Higley, Philip I., 68
Hillman, C. C., 26-27
Hobby, Gladys, 7, 15-16, 30, 34
Hollenberg, Henry, 36-37
Hoover, Herbert, 87
Hull, Cordell, 87, 93
Hutchings, Edward, Jr., 105
Hygienic Institute, 28

I
Insulin, 11-12
Interurban Clinical Club (ICC), 53

J
Johns Hopkins Medical School, 15, 28, 32, 46-50, 52, 55, 104, 110, 167
Jones, James, 15, 187
Justice Department, 148

K
Karl, Barry, 6, 56, 162
Keefer, Chester, 6, 12, 15-17, 31-39, 49-50, 52-53, 55-56, 58-59, 68-93, 103-118, 121-123, 132-134, 137-139, 146, 154-156, 158, 165, 167, 169-172, 175, 185-190, 193
Kidney dialysis, 3, 18, 145, 190
Knowles, Lawrence, 110
Koch, Roy, 168

L
Lewis, Sinclair, 57
Lockwood, John, 27, 32, 51, 53, 79-80, 167, 186
Loewe, Leo, 15-16, 81, 185
Loma Linda Medical Center, 3
Long, Perrin H., 27-28, 30-31, 50, 52-54, 167
Longcope, W. T., 49
Ludmerer, Kenneth, 46-47
Lyme, Harry, 2, 189
Lyons, Champ, 31, 33, 36-38, 51, 105, 121, 154-155, 167

M

MacDonald, H. H., 115
MacFarlane, Gwyn, 7
MacNeal, Ward J., 16, 81, 85, 185
Magazines, 57, 75, 105, 107-112, 114, 119-120, 122, 140-141, 143-145, 154, 156-157, 159, 161, 190
Magee, James, 26, 28, 37
Mahoney, John F., 27, 42
Malone, Patricia, 74-75, 106, 111-112
Maloney, Francis, 86-87
Manhattan Project, 56, 162
Marks, Harry, 11, 27, 55, 78, 85-86, 172-173
Marrow transplants, 3
Marshall, Eli K. Jr., 27, 32, 50, 53-54, 167
Massachusetts General Hospital (MGH), 33, 36, 48, 51, 103
Mayo Clinic, 82-85
McDonell, John N., 138-142
Mechanic, David, 17-18
Media, 2-3, 5, 15-17, 74-77, 103-123, 159-161, 170-172
    advertisements, 118-121, 123
    books, 144-145
    cartoons, 117-118
    magazines, 57, 75, 105, 107-112, 114, 119-120, 122, 140-141, 143-145, 154, 156-157, 159, 161, 190
    motion pictures, 56-58, 103, 115-116, 121
    newspapers, 57, 74-76, 103-115, 123, 163
    newsreels, 115, 122
    radio, 117, 121-122
    television, 3, 190
Meningitis, 145, 170
Mentally ill, 135-137, 146
Mentally retarded, 135, 137, 146, 186
Merck Pharmaceuticals, 9, 34, 38, 122
Middle Georgia Hospital, 106

Moley, Raymond, 56
Motion pictures, 56-58, 103, 115-116, 121
Moyer, Andrew J., 132
Mussey, R. D., 84-85

N

Napoleonic Wars, 10
National ACademy of Sciences, 30
National Cancer Institute (NCI), 165, 167
National Defense Research Committee (NDRC), 6
National Institute of Mental Health (NIMH), 165
National Institutes of Health (NIH), 165
National research Council (NCR), 15, 27, 30, 39, 84, 105, 110
    Division of Medical Sciences (DMS), 6, 25-29, 31, 68, 88, 122
Nelson, Donald, 132
Nelson, William, 14, 66
New Deal, 45, 56, 65, 136
New Haven Hospital, 51
Newspapers, 57, 74-76, 103-115, 123, 163
Newsreels, 115, 122
Noonan, John T., Jr., 9-10, 93
North African campaign, 10-11
Northern Regional Research Laboratory (NRRL), 33, 114, 132
Novels, 56-57

O

Office of Civilian Penicilin Distribution (OCPD), 6, 10-11, 15, 59, 67, 92, 131-146, 167, 172, 185-187
    Task Committee on Civilian Distribution (TCCD), 132-139, 144-146, 186
Office of Civilian Requirements, 134
Office of Emergency Management, 30

Index

Office of Price Administration, 65
Office of Scientific Research and Development (OSRD), 6, 30, 65-66, 69, 71-73, 104, 122, 162
   Committee on Medical Research (CMR), 6, 8, 14, 16-17, 30, 33, 38, 56, 71-73, 82-84, 86, 88, 92, 103-106, 111, 115, 122-123, 134, 193
   Legal Division of, 14, 71, 81, 189
Office of War Information (OWI), 13, 16-17, 103, 115-117, 139
Olitski, Peter, 53
Oppenheimer, Robert, 56
Organ transplants, 2-5, 18, 153-154, 190
   legal aspects of, 66-67
Osteomyelitis, 189

P

Paine, C. G., 7
Parran, Thomas, 74-75, 165-166
Pasteur, Louis, 58
Peabody, Francis, 27, 49, 51-52
Peking Union Medical College (PUMC), 32, 49, 52
Penicillin
   abuse of, 153-154, 156-161
   allergies to, 155-157, 159, 161
   ampicillin, 173
   blackmarket, 131, 133, 144-146
   Bushnell project, 35-38, 51, 69, 105
   development of, 7-9, 29-38
   free market, 142-146
   for greatest good, 67-93
   home-made, 114-115
   manufacture of, 9, 38, 118-120, 131-132
   media coverage of, 15-17, 74-77, 93, 103-12
   rationing of, 5-7, 9-18, 39, 58-59, 66-93, 131-146, 167, 185-190
   rush on, 103-123
   semisynthetic, 173
   tainted, 144-145

Peter Bent Brigham Hospital, 47-48, 51
Pfizer Pharmeceuticals, 15-16, 38, 155
Pharmacies, 140-143
Physicians
   academic, 45-59, 158, 162-173
   practitioners, 46, 55, 134, 146, 157-158, 161, 174-175, 187-188, 190
Pinanski, Jean, 104
Pittsburgh Presbyterian Hospital, 4
Pneumonia, 86, 136, 141, 145
Polenberg, William, 6
Polio, 144
   vaccine for, 167
Potter, Robert D., 111-112
Practitioners, 46, 55, 134, 146, 157-158, 161, 174-175, 187-188, 190
Presbyterian Hospital
   Columbia University, 8, 47, 51
   Pittsburgh, 4
President's Science Advisory Committee on Bioastronautics, 167
Public Health Service, 26, 164-167
Pulmonary infections, 170

Q

Queen, Frank B., 35-38

R

Radio, 117, 121-122
Radio Corporation of America (RCA), 120
Rapaport, Felix T., 5-6
Raper, Kenneth, 114-115, 168
Ratcliff, J. D., 159-160
Rationing, 1
   AZT, 5, 18, 175
   Committee on Chemotherapeutic and Other Agents (COC), 5-7, 10-17, 25-39, 45, 49-61, 66-93, 103-104, 111, 115, 122-123, 131-134, 143-144, 146, 169-176, 185-190

criticism of, 74-93
flaws in, 136-137
for greatest good, 67-93, 186-187
insulin, 11-12
legacy of, 153-176
legal aspects of, 66-67, 71-73, 80-81, 148
lessons from, 185-190
media coverage, 15-17, 74-77, 93, 103-123
Office of Civilian Penicillin Distribution (OCPD), 6, 10-11, 15, 59, 92, 131-146, 167, 172, 185-187
penicillin, 5-7, 9-18, 39, 58-59, 66-93, 131-146, 167, 185-190
polio vaccine, 167
randomized selection, 187-188
during Second World War, 1, 5-7, 13, 64
streptomycin, 17-18, 146, 167-173
Task Committee on Civilian Distribution (TCCD), 132-139, 144-146, 186
Richards, A. N., 8, 16-17, 30-33, 35-39, 71-73, 76, 82-83, 86-88, 103-118, 123, 132, 154, 164
Robinson, Paul, 107
Rockefeller Institute for Medical Research (RIMR), 28, 49, 51-52
Rocky Mountain Spotted Fever, 173
Rogers, David E., 54
Rogers, John G., 112
Roosevelt, Eleanor, 87-91, 186
Roosevelt, Franklin, 56, 87-90, 93, 97, 99, 110, 162
Rosen, George, 47
Rostenberg, Adolph, Jr., 155
Rusco Machine Belts, 119

S

Saint Louis Children's Hospital, 47

Salmonella, 171
Science Advisory Board, 163-164, 180
Scott, Wilson, 114
Second World War, 5-12
  medical preparedness for, 25-39
  North African campaign, 10-11
  rationing during, 1, 5-7, 13, 64
  research during, 6-7, 25-38
Semisynthetic penicillin, 173
Shapiro, Edward, 110-111
Sheehan, John C., 7, 131, 144
Shryock, Richard, 57, 158
Simmons, J. S., 26-27
Smith, Jack, 15
South-Eastern Organ Procurement Foundation, 4
Spanish-American War, 27
Speh, C. F., 108
Spink, Wesley, 31
Squibb, 8-9, 38, 74-75, 120, 155
Staphylococcal infections, 8, 33-35, 70, 114, 136, 144, 149, 154-155
  penicillin resistant, 154
Staphylococcus aureus superinfections, 171
SAtate University of New York's Downstate Medical Center, 167
Steelman, John R., 164-165
Stephenson, C. S., 26, 28, 40
Stock, Fred, 132, 138, 142
Streptococcal infections, 8, 35, 70, 80, 89, 136, 144
Streptomycin, 153, 159-160, 185
  allergies to, 171
  rationing, 17-18, 146, 167-173
Subacute bacterial endocarditis (SBE), 15-16, 78-81, 189
  bacterial endocarditis, 98, 113, 142, 159, 185-186
Subcommittee on Infectious Diseases, 31-32
Subcommittee on Surgical Infections, 36, 51
Sulfadiazine, 34
Sulfaguanidine, 51

Index

Sulfapyridine, 50-51
Sulfonamides, 29-31, 33-35, 42, 50, 70, 87, 104-105, 107, 136, 159, 170
Swan, Harold T., 7
Syphilis, 159, 173, 187

T

Task Committee on Civilian Distribution (TCCD), 132-139, 144-146, 186
Television, 3, 190
Terramycin, 168, 173, 176
Thorndike Laboratory, 27, 32, 48-49, 52
Tuberculosis, 170-171, 186
Tugwell, R. G., 56
Tulane University, 167
Tuleremia, 170
Tuskegee Syphilis Experiment, 187
Tyor, Peter, 137
Typhoid, 171, 173
Typhus, 173

U

Ulcerative colitis, 90-91
United States Department of Agriculture (USDA), 8, 108, 163
  Northern Regional Research Laboratory (NRRL), 33, 114, 132
United States Public Health Service (USPHS), 164-167
University of Chicago, 32
University of Michigan Medical School, 27, 48, 52
University of Minnesota, 51
University of Rochester School of Medicine and Dentistry, 168
Urticaria, 161, 171

V

Vandercook, John, 122
Veterans Administration, 167, 172
Viral respiratory infections, 174
Vogel, Julius, 114

W

Wainwright, Milton, 7
War Industries Board, 13
War Production Board, 13, 39, 59, 65, 67, 69, 82, 92, 107-108, 118, 121, 131-132, 142
  Chemicals Bureau, 138
  Drugs and Cosmetic Branch, 138
War Relocation Authority, 65
Washington University Medical School, 47, 50, 167
Weber, Max, 9
Weed, Lewis H., 25-27, 31-32, 68
Welch, Henry, 155
Westinghouse, 120
White Cross Hospital, 110
Whorton, James, 157, 174
Wiebe, Robert H., 13
Williams, Joe, 4
Winkler, Allan, 116
Winslow, Gerald R., 10
Winthrop Chemicals, 38, 106, 155
Wood, W. Barry, Jr., 32, 49-50, 53-54, 167
World War I, 11-13
  Committee on Public Information, 13, 106
  Division of Medical Sciences (DMS), 25
World War II, 5-12
  medical preparedness for, 25-39
  Northern African campaign, 10-11
  rationing during, 1, 5-7, 13, 64
  research during, 6-7, 25-38
Worthington Air Conditioning, 120
Wright, A. Dickson, 7-8

Y

Yale, 15, 51-52, 167
York Refrigeration and Air Conditioning, 119-120

Z

Zinsser, Hans, 50